T0198193

Topics in Pediatric Transfusion Medicine

Editors

SARAH R. VOSSOUGHI
BRIE A. STOTLER

CLINICS IN LABORATORY MEDICINE

www.labmed.theclinics.com

Editor-in-Chief
MILENKO JOVAN TANASIJEVIC

March 2021 • Volume 41 • Number 1

ELSEVIER

1600 John F. Kennedy Boulevard • Suite 1800 • Philadelphia, Pennsylvania, 19103-2899

http://www.theclinics.com

CLINICS IN LABORATORY MEDICINE Volume 41, Number 1
March 2021 ISSN 0272-2712, ISBN-13: 978-0-323-76314-1

Editor: Katerina Heidhausen
Developmental Editor: Laura Fisher

Reprints. For copies of 100 or more, of articles in this publication, please contact the Commercial Reprints Department, Elsevier Inc., 360 Park Avenue South, New York, New York 10010-1710. Tel. 212-633-3874, Fax: 212-633-3820, E-mail: reprints@elsevier.com.

Clinics in Laboratory Medicine (ISSN 0272-2712) is published quarterly by Elsevier Inc., 360 Park Avenue South, New York, NY 10010-1710. Months of issue are March, June, September, and December. Business and Editorial offices: 1600 John F. Kennedy Blvd., Suite 1800, Philadelphia, PA 19103-2899. Periodicals postage paid at NewYork, NY and additional mailing offices. Subscription prices are $283.00 per year (US individuals), $731.00 per year (US institutions), $100.00 per year (US students), $363.00 per year (Canadian individuals), $768.00 per year (Canadian institutions), $100.00 per year (Canadian students), $404.00 per year (international individuals), $768.00 per year (international institutions), $185.00 (international students). Foreign air speed delivery is included in all Clinics subscription prices. All prices are subject to change without notice. POSTMASTER: Send address changes to *Clinics in Laboratory Medicine*, Elsevier Health Sciences Division, Subscription Customer Service, 3251 Riverport Lane, Maryland Heights, MO 63043. **Customer Service: 1-800-654-2452 (US). From outside of the US and Canada, call 1-314-447-8871. Fax: 1-314-447-8029. E-mail: journalscustomerservice-usa@elsevier.com (for print support) or journalsonlinesupport-usa@elsevier.com (for online support).**

Clinics in Laboratory Medicine is covered in *EMBASE/Exerpta Medica, MEDLINE/PubMed (Index Medicus), Cinahl, Current Contents/Clinical Medicine, BIOSIS and ISI/BIOMED.*

Printed in the United States of America.

Contributors

EDITOR-IN-CHIEF

MILENKO JOVAN TANASIJEVIC, MD, MBA
Vice Chair for Clinical Pathology and Quality, Department of Pathology, Director of Clinical Laboratories, Brigham and Women's Hospital, Dana-Farber Cancer Institute, Associate Professor of Pathology, Harvard Medical School, Boston, Massachusetts, USA

EDITORS

SARAH R. VOSSOUGHI, MD, RN
Assistant Professor, Department of Pathology and Cell Biology, Columbia University Irving Medical Center, New York, New York, USA

BRIE A. STOTLER, MD, MPH
Associate Professor, Department of Pathology and Cell Biology, Columbia University Irving Medical Center, New York, New York, USA

AUTHORS

JENNIFER ANDREWS, MD, MSc
Associate Professor, Department of Pathology, Microbiology and Immunology, Division of Transfusion Medicine, Department of Pediatrics, Division of Hematology/Oncology, Vanderbilt University Medical Center, Nashville, Tennessee, USA

KYLE ANNEN, DO
Assistant Professor, Department of Pathology, University of Colorado Anschutz Medical Campus, Medical Director of Transfusion Services and Patient Blood Management, Department of Pathology and Laboratory Medicine, Children's Hospital Colorado, Aurora, Colorado, USA

JILLIAN M. BAKER, MD, MSc, FRCPC
Assistant Professor of Pediatrics, University of Toronto, Pediatric Hematologist, Unity Health Toronto (St. Michael's Hospital), The Hospital for Sick Children, Toronto, Ontario, Canada

MICHAEL AARON BECKWITH, MD
Division of Trauma and Acute Care Surgery, Assistant Professor, Department of Surgery, The University of Alabama at Birmingham, Birmingham, Alabama, USA

JEREMY W. CANNON, MD, MA, FACS
Division of Traumatology, Surgical Critical Care, and Emergency Surgery, Associate Professor, Department of Surgery, University of Pennsylvania Perelman School of Medicine, Penn Presbyterian Medical Center, Philadelphia, Pennsylvania, USA

STELLA T. CHOU, MD
Associate Professor of Pediatrics, Department of Pediatrics, The Children's Hospital of Philadelphia, University of Pennsylvania School of Medicine, Philadelphia, Pennsylvania, USA

MEGHAN DELANEY, DO, MPH
Chief, Pathology and Laboratory Medicine Division, Director, Transfusion Medicine, Children's National Hospital, Professor of Pathology and Pediatrics, The George Washington University, Washington, DC, USA

MELKON DOMBOURIAN, MD
Assistant Professor, Department of Pathology, University of Colorado Anschutz Medical Campus, Medical Director of Network of Care Laboratories, Main Core Laboratory and Point of Care Testing, Department of Pathology and Laboratory Medicine, Associate Medical Director of Transfusion Services and Patient Blood Management, Children's Hospital Colorado, Aurora, Colorado, USA

HYOJEONG HAN, MD
Blood Bank Fellow, Pathology and Immunology, Baylor College of Medicine, Houston, Texas, USA

JEANNE E. HENDRICKSON, MD
Professor, Departments of Laboratory Medicine and Pediatrics, Yale University, New Haven, Connecticut, USA

LISA HENSCH, MD
Assistant Professor, Pathology and Immunology, Baylor College of Medicine, Houston, Texas, USA

SHIU-KI ROCKY HUI, MD
Associate Professor, Pathology and Immunology and Pediatrics, Baylor College of Medicine, Houston, Texas, USA

MELANIE E. JACKSON, MBBS, BSc, DCH
Pediatric Hematology Sub-Specialty Fellow, The Hospital for Sick Children, Toronto, Ontario, Canada

CASSANDRA D. JOSEPHSON, MD
Professor, Department of Laboratory Medicine and Pathology, Center for Transfusion Medicine and Cellular Therapies, Department of Pediatrics, Aflac Cancer and Blood Disorders Center, Emory University School of Medicine, Atlanta, Georgia, USA

SUSAN KULDANEK, MD
Instructor, Hemophilia and Thrombosis Center, Center for Cancer and Blood Disorders, Children's Hospital Colorado, University of Colorado Anschutz Medical Campus, Aurora, Colorado, USA

YUNCHUAN DELORES MO, MD, MSC
Associate Medical Director, Transfusion Medicine, Children's National Hospital, Assistant Professor of Pathology and Pediatrics, The George Washington University, Washington, DC, USA

LUCAS P. NEFF, MD, FACS
Assistant Professor, Department of General Surgery, Section of Pediatric Surgery, Wake Forest University School of Medicine, Winston-Salem, North Carolina, USA

BRYCE PASKO, MD
Assistant Professor, Department of Pathology and Laboratory Medicine, Children's Hospital Colorado, Department of Pathology, University of Colorado Anschutz Medical Campus, Aurora, Colorado, USA

JENNA T. REECE, MD
Pathology and Laboratory Medicine, University of Pennsylvania Perelman School of Medicine, Transfusion Medicine Fellow, The Hospital of the University of Pennsylvania, Philadelphia, Pennsylvania, USA

ROBERT T. RUSSELL, MD, MPH
Division of Pediatric Surgery, Associate Professor, Department of Surgery, The University of Alabama at Birmingham, Birmingham, Alabama, USA

DEBORAH SESOK-PIZZINI, MD, MBA
Professor of Clinical Pathology and Laboratory Medicine, University of Pennsylvania Perelman School of Medicine, The Children's Hospital of Philadelphia, Philadelphia, Pennsylvania, USA

NATALIYA SOSTIN, MD, MCR
Assistant Professor, Department of Laboratory Medicine, Yale University, New Haven, Connecticut, USA

PHILIP C. SPINELLA, MD, FCCM
Division of Critical Care Medicine, Professor, Department of Pediatrics, Washington University in St. Louis, St Louis, Missouri, USA

JUN TERUYA, MD, DSc
Professor, Pathology and Immunology, Pediatrics, and Medicine, Baylor College of Medicine, Houston, Texas, USA

SHANNON C. WALKER, MD
Fellow, Department of Pediatrics, Division of Hematology/Oncology, Vanderbilt University Medical Center, Nashville, Tennessee, USA

PATRICIA E. ZERRA, MD
Assistant Professor, Department of Laboratory Medicine and Pathology, Center for Transfusion Medicine and Cellular Therapies, Department of Pediatrics, Aflac Cancer and Blood Disorders Center, Emory University School of Medicine, Atlanta, Georgia, USA

YAN ZHENG, MD, PhD
Assistant Member, Department of Pathology, St. Jude Children's Research Hospital, Memphis, Tennessee, USA

Contents

> Children require transfusion of blood components for a vast array of medical conditions, including acute hemorrhage, hematologic and nonhematologic malignancies, hemoglobinopathy, and allogeneic and autologous stem cell transplant. Evidence-based literature on pediatric transfusion practices is limited, particularly for non–red blood cell products, and many recommendations are extrapolated from studies in adult populations. Recognition of these knowledge gaps has led to increasing numbers of clinical trials focusing on children and establishment of pediatric transfusion working groups in recent years. This article reviews existing literature on pediatric transfusion therapy within the larger context of analogous data in adult populations.

> Transfusion of red blood cells, platelets, and fresh frozen plasma in neonatal patients has not been well characterized in the literature, with guidelines varying greatly between institutions. However, anemia and thrombocytopenia are highly prevalent, especially in preterm neonates. When transfusing a neonatal patient, clinicians must take into consideration physiologic differences, gestational and postnatal age, congenital disorders, and maternal factors while weighing the risks and benefits of transfusion. This review of existing literature summarizes current evidence-based neonatal transfusion guidelines and highlights areas of current ongoing research and those in need of future studies.

> Massive transfusion in pediatric patients is infrequent but associated with much higher mortality than in adults. Blood transfusion and hematology has conceptualized ideas such as blood failure and the interplay of the blood-endothelium interface to understand coagulopathy in the context of hemorrhagic shock. Researchers are still searching for an appropriate definition of what constitutes a pediatric massive transfusion. There is no universally accepted protocol for massive transfusion and how to address the many complications that can arise. Pharmacologic adjuncts to resuscitation may prove beneficial in reducing coagulopathy during pediatric massive transfusion, but high-quality evidence has not yet emerged.

Some types of transfusion reactions occur more frequently in the pediatric than the adult population. Allergic reactions are the most common, followed by nonhemolytic transfusion reactions; male children seem most susceptible to such reactions. Platelets are often implicated and pulmonary reactions are understudied in children. Clinical sequelae in neonates, such as bronchopulmonary dysplasia/chronic lung disease and intraventricular hemorrhage, have received increasing attention in relation to transfusion. There is a need to better understand the pathophysiology of transfusion reactions in neonatal and pediatric populations so preventive strategies can be undertaken. There is also a need for robust hemovigilance systems.

Blood banks need to understand patterns of use and ordering practices to provide the blood donor centers with the best information with which to develop daily scheduled deliveries of blood products. Blood use is a large component of this process through maximizing physician education about appropriate ordering practices and use of appropriate tools. Simple measures can help provide guidance on the number of available components and the need to order more from the blood donor center. Special product requests in pediatrics, such as fresh blood, leukoreduction, irradiation, and antigen-negative units can also drive inventory practices and use patterns.

The diagnosis of coagulopathy or thrombophilia in pediatric patients can be challenging. Congenital coagulopathies often present in the pediatric period and require appropriate work-up for diagnosis and ongoing management. Acquired coagulopathies of childhood are frequently encountered in hospitalized children and warrant appropriate coagulation testing for goal-directed therapy. The incidence of thrombosis is increasing in pediatric patients. After identifying the presence of thrombus, acute management includes initiating therapeutic anticoagulation. Choice of anticoagulant depends on patient's clinical status, along with availability of the anticoagulant. Thrombophilia evaluation is performed when children present with spontaneous thrombosis. Thrombophilia tests are inaccurate during acute illness.

Red blood cell (RBC) transfusion is critical in managing acute and chronic complications of sickle cell disease. Alloimmunization and iron overload remain significant complications of transfusion therapy and are minimized with prophylactic Rh and K antigen RBC matching and iron chelation. Matched sibling donor hematopoietic stem cell transplant (HSCT) is a curative therapeutic option. Autologous hematopoietic stem cell (HSC)–based gene therapy has recently shown great promise, for which obtaining sufficient HSCs is essential for success. This article discusses RBC transfusion indications and complications, transfusion support during HSCT, and HSC mobilization and collection for autologous HSCT with gene therapy.

Topics in Pediatric Transfusion Medicine
CLINICS IN LABORATORY MEDICINE

SERIES OF RELATED INTEREST

Surgical Pathology Clinics
Available at: https://www.surgpath.theclinics.com/

THE CLINICS ARE NOW AVAILABLE ONLINE!
Access your subscription at:
www.theclinics.com

Preface

The Development of the Nascent Field of Pediatric Transfusion Medicine

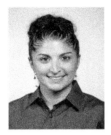
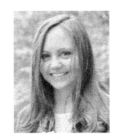

Sarah R. Vossoughi, MD, RN   Brie A. Stotler, MD, MPH
Editors

The concept of childhood is a more recent construct of civilization from the seventeenth century. Previously in human history, once a person could walk and talk, there was no distinction, and more importantly, no protection for this vulnerable time in development. This transition in thinking of childhood as a distinct entity separate from adulthood with distinct developmental stages and special needs gave birth to the specialty of pediatrics in the late nineteenth century. There is now worldwide recognition of the special status of children in many cultures, and we are just beginning to understand the depth of these differences, which are potentially greater than anyone could have predicted. As the concepts of childhood and adulthood have continued to evolve, children are now known to have unique health considerations, distinct diseases, and even different biochemical profiles from adults. In transfusion medicine, emerging evidence has continued to show that the principles once applied universally to all ages cannot be extrapolated to children by simply adjusting for smaller total blood volumes. The past several decades have explored concepts from which additive solutions are safe in children all the way to more recent explorations into emerging cellular therapies for childhood diseases once thought to be incurable, such as sickle cell disease. The arena of pediatric transfusion medicine continues to gain momentum and produce a body of research expanding at an astounding pace. This issue of *Clinics in Laboratory Medicine* covers the current evidence-based guidelines, hemovigilance, product selection, coagulation, cellular therapies, hemolytic disease of the fetus and newborn, and novel blood component therapies for the pediatric and neonatal patient. With this special issue, we hope to summarize some of the most recent research,

Clin Lab Med 41 (2021) xi–xii
https://doi.org/10.1016/j.cll.2020.12.001
0272-2712/21/© 2020 Published by Elsevier Inc.   labmed.theclinics.com

review the current understanding of best practices, and touch on what to expect in the future from the leading experts in this exciting field.

Sarah R. Vossoughi, MD, RN
Department of Pathology and Cell Biology
Columbia University Irving Medical Center
Harkness Pavilion, Room 4-425B
622 West 168th Street
New York, NY 10032, USA

Brie A. Stotler, MD, MPH
Department of Pathology and Cell Biology
Columbia University Irving Medical Center
Harkness Pavilion, Room 4-414
622 West 168th Street
New York, NY 10032, USA

E-mail addresses:
sv2473@cumc.columbia.edu (S.R. Vossoughi)
bs2277@cumc.columbia.edu (B.A. Stotler)

Transfusion in Pediatric Patients
Review of Evidence-Based Guidelines

Yunchuan Delores Mo, MD, MSC[a],*, Meghan Delaney, DO, MPH[b]

KEYWORDS

- Pediatric • Transfusion threshold • Evidence-based • Red blood cells • Platelets
- Plasma

KEY POINTS

- Pediatric transfusion practices are highly variable because of the limited amount of evidence-based literature and challenges surrounding development and implementation of standardized guidelines.
- A restrictive red blood cell transfusion threshold of 7 g/dL is generally considered to be safe for stable, nonbleeding, critically ill children.
- Recommended platelet transfusion thresholds for adults may not be appropriate in pediatric populations because children seem to have a higher risk of clinically significant bleeding independent of platelet count.
- Prophylactic plasma transfusion in children is not effective for correction of mild coagulopathy and unnecessarily increases the risk of transfusion-related adverse events.

INTRODUCTION

Transfusion therapy represents a valuable treatment modality for a variety of medical conditions, including acute blood loss and selective deficiency of 1 or more cell lines. Because most blood components cannot be synthetically manufactured, they represent a finite and limited resource that must be wisely used, especially because the United States and other countries largely rely on volunteer blood donors. Indications for the use of blood components have evolved over the last half century with increasing emphasis placed on practices rooted in firm scientific principles in recent decades. To this end, numerous studies have been conducted in order to expand this database and optimize transfusion therapy in various patient populations. Several

[a] Transfusion Medicine, Children's National Hospital, 111 Michigan Avenue Northwest, Laboratory Administration, Suite 2100, Washington, DC 20010, USA; [b] Pathology and Laboratory Medicine Division, Transfusion Medicine, Children's National Hospital, 111 Michigan Avenue Northwest, Laboratory Administration, Suite 2100, Washington, DC 20010, USA
* Corresponding author.
E-mail address: ymo@childrensnational.org

Clin Lab Med 41 (2021) 1–14
https://doi.org/10.1016/j.cll.2020.10.001 **labmed.theclinics.com**
0272-2712/21/© 2020 Elsevier Inc. All rights reserved.

notable randomized controlled trials investigating liberal versus restrictive red blood cell (RBC) transfusion thresholds[1,2] have proved to be particularly influential in changing clinical perceptions. These studies have led to the development of evidence-based transfusion guidelines in adult populations. Patient blood management (PBM) initiatives promote adherence to such guidelines and emphasize assessment of both the risks and benefits of blood product use before transfusion.[3] Establishment of similar guidelines for pediatric patients has been challenging because of the paucity of data from rigorous studies and hesitation associated with conducting research on vulnerable patient populations. Although increased awareness of the knowledge gaps has driven further research, a significant number of pediatric transfusion practices are still based on historical or anecdotal data or are derived from data extrapolated from adult populations. This article provides an overview of the evidence available to date regarding pediatric transfusion guidelines.

RED BLOOD CELLS

A large proportion of the literature on pediatric transfusion indications is focused on RBC transfusion. RBCs are indicated for treatment of blood loss and acute or chronic anemia in order to increase hemoglobin levels and restore adequate oxygen carrying capacity and tissue perfusion.[4] For patients with hemoglobinopathies such as sickle cell disease, chronic transfusion therapy is also used to prevent complications resulting from the presence of abnormal hemoglobin variants. The decision to transfuse RBCs is multifactorial, including consideration of hemoglobin/hematocrit levels or other laboratory values, clinical presentation (ie, signs and symptoms of anemia), patient age and physiology, and underlying medical status. Although RBC transfusion is generally recommended for children experiencing acute blood loss exceeding 15% to 20% of their total blood volume,[5] the decision ultimately depends on individual patient characteristics. The therapeutic benefits of administering blood components must be weighed against the risks, including adverse events such as acute and delayed transfusion reactions, alloimmunization, physiologic derangements (eg, hyperkalemia, hypothermia), and exposure to allogeneic blood. Alternative therapies such as iron supplementation and other blood conservation strategies should also be considered if medically appropriate.[6]

Randomized controlled trials (RCTs) have aimed to elucidate the ideal hemoglobin trigger for RBC transfusion. In 1999, the Transfusion Requirements in Critical Care (TRICC) trial[1] showed that nonbleeding, critically ill adult patients subjected to a restrictive transfusion threshold of 7 g/dL seemed to have lower mortalities and fewer cardiopulmonary complications compared with similar patients randomized to a liberal threshold of 10 g/dL. Following that publication, the Transfusion Requirements in the Pediatric Intensive Care Unit (TRIPICU) study[7] compared restrictive (7 g/dL) versus liberal (9.5 g/dL) transfusion thresholds in hemodynamically stable, critically ill children admitted to the pediatric intensive care unit (PICU). The investigators enrolled a total of 637 subjects, randomizing 320 to the restrictive strategy arm and 317 to the liberal strategy arm, and evaluated primary outcomes characterized by severity and/or progression of multiorgan dysfunction syndrome. They also studied secondary outcomes such as 28-day mortality, length of stay, sepsis, transfusion reactions, and infection rates. No statistically significant differences were detected in the 2 groups for any of the outcomes. There was no evidence of excess harm or adverse events occurring in patients in the restrictive arm. Unlike adults in the liberal study arm of the TRICC trial, patients in the TRIPICU liberal group did not have increased mortality or cardiopulmonary complications. The investigators attributed this difference between adults and children to possible increased vulnerability to detrimental effects of transfusion in the former and differential availability of prestorage leukocyte-reduced components. The TRIPICU study investigators noted that patients in the restrictive arm had a 96% reduction in any transfusion exposure and a 44% decrease in administered RBC transfusions compared with the liberal group. Subgroup analyses of TRIPICU patients with severe illness, sepsis, noncyanotic cardiac disease or after cardiac surgery, respiratory dysfunction, acute lung injury, neurologic dysfunction, and severe trauma continued to support a restrictive transfusion threshold of 7 g/dL, although there was insufficient evidence for cyanotic patients.[8] The results of a smaller RCT suggested that children with single-ventricle physiology might benefit from a slightly higher restrictive threshold of 9 g/dL (compared with 13 g/dL for the liberal arm).[9] Although pediatric intensivists have largely agreed that patients in hemorrhagic shock require transfusion, consensus about the amount of RBCs to transfuse has not been reached.[8] Hemoglobin thresholds are less useful in the setting of acute hemorrhage because significant losses can occur before detection via laboratory values, although nadir levels of 5 g/dL have been proposed as an absolute lower limit for critically ill patients.[10] In the absence of prospective clinical trials studying clinically unstable children who are not in hemorrhagic or septic shock, general recommendations include reliance on clinical judgment or goal-directed therapy with physiologic targets (eg, central venous O_2 saturation).[8]

Subsequent RCTs have largely shown that restrictive transfusion strategies can be safely applied in adults with septic shock,[11] acute gastrointestinal hemorrhage,[12,13] traumatic brain injury,[14] and cardiac[15,16] and oncologic[17] surgical intervention. Large-scale meta-analyses of adult and (limited) pediatric trials did not detect benefits resulting from liberal transfusion, nor increased morbidity or mortality associated with use of restrictive thresholds.[18,19] Several clinical practice guidelines published since these trials have fully endorsed a restrictive approach.[20,21] In their most recent RBC guidelines, the AABB (formerly known as the American Association of Blood Banks) recommended transfusion thresholds of 7 g/dL for hemodynamically stable inpatients and 8 g/dL for patients with prior cardiovascular disease or those undergoing cardiac or orthopedic surgery instead of the previous standard threshold of 10 g/dL.[22] They refrained from making recommendations for outpatients or those with acute coronary syndrome, hematologic or oncologic disorders, severe thrombocytopenia, or chronic transfusion-dependent anemia because of insufficient evidence. The British Committee for Standards in Haematology (BCSH) published an update[23] of their previous pediatric guidelines[24] in which they recommended thresholds of 7 g/dL for stable, noncyanotic PICU patients or perioperative patients undergoing noncardiac surgery and 7 to 8 g/dL for pediatric stem cell and oncology patients based on limited pediatric[25] and adult[26] evidence. In keeping with PBM initiatives to limit RBC transfusion to a single unit at a time in nonbleeding adults, the group also recommended minimizing transfusion volumes in children by limiting the posttransfusion increment to a maximum of 2 g/dL above the recommended hemoglobin threshold (typically equivalent to a maximum of 1 unit for an adult).[23]

In 2018, participants in the Pediatric Critical Care Transfusion and Anemia Expertise Initiative (TAXI) published RBC transfusion guidelines based on available evidence or expert consensus when evidence was lacking.[27] In addition to recommendations aimed toward a general population of critically ill children,[28] they provided separate recommendations for 8 other diagnostic categories, including (1) acute respiratory failure[29]; (2) nonhemorrhagic shock[30]; (3) non–life-threatening bleeding and hemorrhagic shock[31]; (4) acute brain injury[32]; (5) acquired and congenital heart disease[33]; (6) sickle cell and oncologic disease[34]; (7) support from extracorporeal circuit membrane oxygenation (ECMO), ventricular assist devices, and renal replacement therapy[35]; and (8) use of alternative processing of blood products.[36] The recommendations provided for the general population of critically ill children incorporated previously published guidelines by incorporating 5 g/dL as the minimum and 7 g/dL as the maximum transfusion thresholds in hemodynamically stable patients.[27,28] They were unable to provide specific recommendations when hemoglobin levels ranged from 5 to 7 g/dL and advocated the use of clinical judgment in such situations. Other TAXI recommendations advised targeting posttransfusion hemoglobin levels of 7 to 9.5 g/dL rather than attempting to correct levels into the normal range for age. Despite discussion of specific hemoglobin thresholds, the investigators emphasized the need for careful consideration of the patient's overall clinical context rather than relying solely on select laboratory values. Many of the general recommendations were applicable to patients in the other subgroups, although there was often insufficient evidence for specific populations, such as patients with respiratory failure complicated by acute hypoxemia,[29] unstable nonhemorrhagic shock,[30] and pulmonary hypertension with normal cardiac structure.[33] For certain clinical subgroups, the investigators recommended alternative hemoglobin thresholds, such as 7 to 10 g/dL in the setting of acute brain injury,[32] 7 to 8 g/dL for stem cell transplant and oncology patients,[34] and 9 g/dL as a maximum threshold for those with uncorrected cardiac defect or single-ventricle physiology.[33] For patients with life-threatening bleeding, TAXI recommended empiric transfusions of RBCs, plasma, and platelets in a 1:1:1 or 2:1:1 ratio for resuscitation regardless of laboratory values.[31] In the course of evaluating the available evidence, the group also formulated research recommendations to be addressed by future clinical trials, such as investigation of physiologic metrics and biomarkers to guide transfusion therapy in all subpopulations.[27] Systematic reviews of platelet and plasma transfusion indications in critically ill children by the TAXI–Control/Avoidance of Bleeding (CAB) working group are currently ongoing, and recommendations will be presented in a forthcoming publication (M. Delaney, personal communication; 2020).

PLATELETS

Platelet transfusions are indicated for restoring primary hemostasis during hemorrhage as well as prevention of bleeding in the presence of severe thrombocytopenia or acquired or congenital platelet dysfunction.[4] Most transfusions are administered prophylactically to oncologic and hematopoietic stem cell transplant (HSCT) patients with hypoproliferative thrombocytopenia induced by chemotherapy, radiation, or myeloablation.[37,38]

Platelet counts have historically been used as a surrogate marker for determining the likelihood of bleeding. Recent studies in preterm neonates have suggested that restrictive prophylactic thresholds as low as 25,000/μL are safe and may be associated with a lower risk of major bleeding and mortality than more liberal thresholds of greater than 50,000/μL.[39,40] The concern for bleeding in the early neonatal period centers around intraventricular hemorrhage, which may have a different mechanism than bleeding associated with hypoproliferative thrombocytopenia and does not seem to depend on platelet count (Patricia E. Zerra and Cassandra Josephson's article, "Transfusion in the Neonatal Patient: Review of Evidence Based Guidelines," discussed elsewhere in this issue). In pediatric patients, there are few platelet trigger RCTs available to formulate evidence-based recommendations. The 2015 AABB clinical guidelines recommend a transfusion threshold of 10,000/μL to prevent spontaneous hemorrhage in adults with therapy-induced hypoproliferative thrombocytopenia; higher thresholds of 20,000/μL are recommended for those undergoing central venous catheter (CVC) placement and 50,000/μL for lumbar puncture (LP) or major non–central nervous system (CNS) surgery.[41] The extent to which these guidelines may be applied to children is controversial, especially considering evidence of poor correlation between platelet count and bleeding risk in children.[42] Surveys of pediatric intensive care,[38] oncology,[43] and HSCT[44] transfusion practices have revealed highly divergent platelet transfusion thresholds, often at levels significantly greater than recommended prophylactic guidelines (up to 50,000/μL). Several pediatric clinical guidelines recommend a standard transfusion threshold of 5000 to 10,000/μL for stable, nonbleeding children, excluding patients with immune-mediated thrombocytopenia or stable aplastic anemia.[5,23] No definitive guidelines have been established for bleeding or unstable pediatric patients or those with qualitative platelet dysfunction, although higher values (eg, 100,000/μL) or clinical evidence of hemostasis may be targeted in these situations.[21]

The largest prospective randomized transfusion study to include a significant pediatric population is the Optimal Platelet Dose Strategy to Prevent Bleeding in Thrombocytopenia (PLADO) study, which examined the effect of different platelet doses on the incidence of bleeding in 1272 patients with hypoproliferative thrombocytopenia.[45] Patients were randomized to 3 different groups and received low ($1.1 \times 10^{11}/m^2$ of body surface area), medium ($2.2 \times 10^{11}/m^2$), or high ($4.4 \times 10^{11}/m^2$) platelet doses whenever their morning platelet counts were 10,000/μL or less. Although a direct correlation was noted between the dose of platelets given and the incremental response after transfusion (resulting in increased numbers of transfusions in the low dose group), no differences in bleeding outcomes were noted with the doses used in the study. Subgroup analysis of the 200 children who received at least 1 platelet transfusion also did not show an association between platelet dose and incidence of significant bleeding.[42] Notably, the PLADO study found that pediatric patients (aged 0–18 years), particularly those undergoing autologous or syngeneic stem cell transplant, had a significantly higher risk (and increased frequency) of World Health Organization (WHO) grade 2 or higher bleeding compared with adults (aged ≥19 years). This difference was observed regardless of pretransfusion platelet count and suggests that other variables account for the higher incidence of bleeding in children compared with adults, possibly caused by differences in endothelial structure or treatment chemotherapy dose/intensity.[42,46]

Additional studies have explored whether prophylactic transfusions are necessary.[47,48] Two recent RCTs compared a therapeutic approach of transfusing platelets only for clinically significant bleeding (WHO grade 2 or higher) against a prophylactic approach of transfusing platelets when morning counts were less than or equal to 10,000/μL in hematologic malignancy and HSCT patients.[49,50] As expected, the therapeutic group experienced increased frequency of bleeding compared with the prophylactic group, although most were classified as minor bleeds (grade 2) and responded well to platelet transfusion. In 1 study,[49] patients with acute myeloid leukemia (AML) in the therapeutic arm were more likely to have major CNS bleeds (WHO grade 4) compared with autologous HSCT patients, which led the investigators to conclude that autologous stem cell transplant patients could possibly be managed by therapeutic transfusions alone, but that a prophylactic threshold of 10,000/μL should remain the standard of care for patients with AML. The Trial of Prophylactic Platelets (TOPPS) study also showed that oncology/allogeneic HSCT patients experienced greater reduction in bleeding complications than autologous HSCT patients receiving prophylaxis, suggesting that nonautologous HSCT patients benefit more from transfusions administered solely for prevention of bleeding.[51] Based on these findings, the investigators concluded that prophylactic transfusions play an important role in prevention of clinically significant bleeding in patients with hematologic malignancy. In their updated clinical practice guidelines, the American Society of Clinical Oncology (ASCO) recommended continued use of prophylactic transfusions for patients with hematologic malignancies and cautiously endorsed a no-prophylaxis approach in adult (but not pediatric) autologous HSCT recipients.[52]

Platelet transfusion thresholds for patients undergoing invasive procedures[53] or surgery[54] have also been the focus of multiple studies, although conclusive triggers have not been established in patients of any age. A retrospective review of 5223 LPs performed on 958 children with acute lymphoblastic leukemia (ALL) did not find increased rates of bleeding or other major adverse events in severely thrombocytopenic patients (742 LPs performed at platelet count of 21,000–50,000/μL, 170 at 11,000–20,000/μL, and 29 at $\leq$10,000/μL).[55] Based on these findings, the investigators did not recommend prophylactic platelet transfusion before LP for patients with counts greater than 10,000/μL, a far lower safe threshold than the 50,000/μL recommended by AABB for adults.[41] However, other reports seem to indicate higher relapse and lower survival rates for patients with ALL who experience a traumatic LP in the presence of circulating blasts (eg, initial leukemic presentation).[46,56] In order to avoid increased risk of LP-related bleeding in such patients, higher preprocedural thresholds between 50,000[37] and 100,000/μL[57] have been proposed.

AABB[41] and ASCO[52] guidelines recommend a transfusion threshold of 20,000/μL for minor invasive procedures such as bone marrow aspiration/biopsy and CVC insertion. Evidence for the latter was derived from a retrospective review of 604 line placements in 193 adults.[58] For major, non-CNS surgery in patients without bleeding or coagulopathy, ASCO provides a range of 40,000 to 50,000/μL, whereas AABB recommends a minimum count of 50,000/μL. AABB specifically counsels against preprocedural prophylactic platelet transfusion in patients with normal platelet counts undergoing cardiovascular bypass surgery because of an absence of supporting evidence. British practice guidelines[21,23] have proposed 75,000 to 100,000/μL as targets for patients with disseminated intravascular coagulation (DIC) or those undergoing neurologic or ophthalmic surgery. ECMO patients are also heavily transfused because they are systemically heparinized and often experience rapid consumption and activation of circulating platelets by the extracorporeal circuit. Thus, they may require maintenance of counts at 100,000/μL or higher to prevent bleeding complications.[5,38] These pediatric population groups do not have well-powered clinical trials to form the foundation for evidence-based recommendations at this time.

PLASMA

Plasma products include fresh frozen plasma, plasma frozen within 24 hours after phlebotomy, thawed plasma, and solvent-detergent–treated plasma. Most products are used interchangeably in most clinical settings[59] and are collectively referred to as plasma products.[4] Evidence-based indications for plasma transfusion include repletion of multiple coagulation factors during acute hemorrhage in combination with RBCs and platelets as part of a resuscitation protocol[60]; perioperative blood loss; or multifactor deficiency associated with DIC or other consumptive coagulopathies, liver disease,[5] or systemic anticoagulation (eg, ECMO).[61,62] Plasma may also be used for replacement of specific coagulation factors secondary to congenital or acquired deficiencies that are not available as factor concentrates (eg, factor V), reconstitution of whole blood for extracorporeal circuit primes or exchange transfusions, or as replacement fluid for therapeutic plasma exchange in patients with thrombotic thrombocytopenic purpura or other indications complicated by bleeding or coagulopathy.[63] Plasma was historically used for urgent reversal of vitamin K antagonists, although prothrombin complex concentrates are now widely used because of their greater efficacy and safety profile in volume-sensitive patients.[64,65]

Prophylactic plasma transfusions are frequently administered to correct abnormal coagulation parameters such as prolonged prothrombin time (PT), international normalized ratio (INR), or activated partial thromboplastin time (aPTT) in nonbleeding patients before invasive procedures or surgery. The rationale is based on the following central tenets: (1) abnormal coagulation parameters (PT-INR, aPTT) are associated with increased bleeding risk, (2) plasma transfusion is effective in correcting the abnormalities, and (3) normalization of coagulation values results in decreased risk of hemorrhage.[66] These assumptions are problematic because of the inherent limitations of using in vitro assays to assess in vivo thrombosis and maintaining physiologic levels of coagulation factors in exogenous blood products, but they remain prevalent in clinical practice.

Although plasma transfusions are administered to nearly 3% of all pediatric inpatients in the United States[67] and 12% to 13% of all intensive care patients,[68,69] much of the evidence supporting common practices is either absent or of low quality. Multiple RCTs published since the 1970s have failed to show clear indications for plasma administration for either therapeutic or prophylactic purposes in adults and children.[70,71] Expert consensus recommendations have specifically stated that prophylactic plasma transfusions should not be given solely for correction of mild to moderate coagulopathy without active bleeding or planned invasive procedures or surgery.[21,23,63] In spite of the existence of national guidelines in countries such as the United Kingdom and Canada, clinical practices remain idiosyncratic and reflect significant deviations from published recommendations.[72,73] Both adult[74] and pediatric[75] studies have found that more than 65% of plasma transfusions in critically ill patients did not adhere to published guidelines, with approximately 34% of plasma orders being requested for nonbleeding patients without planned invasive procedures. These findings are highly concerning when considering transfusion-related risks and adverse events, as shown by recent studies finding increased organ dysfunction, nosocomial infections,[76] hypercoagulability,[77] and overall mortality associated with plasma transfusions in critically ill children.

The studies referenced earlier also unveiled widely divergent INR thresholds[75] used in various clinical scenarios to guide transfusion decision making, including INR less than 1.5.[69,72,73] An international multicenter prospective study of critically ill pediatric patients examined incremental changes in coagulation parameters and found the differences between pretransfusion and posttransfusion INR (median, 1.5 vs 1.4) and aPTT (median, 48 vs 41 seconds) to be negligible regardless of dose except in cases of severe coagulopathy (INR>2.5 or aPTT>60 seconds).[78] These observations are similar to those previously described in adult or general populations[69,79,80] and confirm that traditional laboratory coagulation values are not sensitive biomarkers for evaluating response to plasma transfusion or for predicting bleeding risks in children with mild coagulopathy.[69] Hemorrhagic complications during invasive procedures, including pediatric liver biopsy[81] and CVC placement,[82] are rare in the setting of mild PT-INR abnormalities (range, 1.5–2.0). A 2005 meta-analysis reviewed the safety profile of various invasive interventions, including bronchoscopy, central vein cannulation, femoral angiography, liver biopsy, kidney biopsy, and other minor procedures.[83] Most did not seem to be associated with increased bleeding, although there were insufficient data for particular procedures (kidney biopsy, LP, and paracentesis and thoracentesis), and the studies were of variable quality overall with inconsistent characterization of the degree of coagulopathy. In the absence of conclusive evidence, expert recommendations in this area are likely to be included in the up-coming TAXI-CAB guidelines.

CRYOPRECIPITATE

Cryoprecipitate is primarily used for fibrinogen replenishment in current clinical prac-tice, although historically it served as a source of factor VIII, von Willebrand factor, and factor XIII before the advent of pharmacologic factor concentrates.[4,5,61,63] Indications include hypofibrinogenemia or dysfibrinogenemia complicated by bleeding (eg, DIC) or prophylaxis before invasive procedures or surgery.[4] Although plasma is also a sig-nificant source of fibrinogen, the much smaller relative volume of cryoprecipitate (10–15 mL vs 200–250 mL of plasma) allows delivery of a concentrated equivalent dose and is an important consideration when transfusing pediatric or volume-sensitive pa-tients.[5] Human-derived (and pathogen-reduced) fibrinogen concentrate is approved for treatment of bleeding episodes in patients with congenital fibrinogen deficiency (ie, afibrinogenemia or hypofibrinogenemia),[84] but is increasingly being used as an alternative to cryoprecipitate for acquired deficiencies. Several RCTs have found fibrinogen concentrate to be equally effective in treating hypofibrinogenemia-related bleeding following cardiac surgery in infants,[85] children,[86] and adults.[87] Massive transfusion protocols have variably incorporated cryoprecipitate or fibrinogen concen-trate, particularly for resuscitation in cases of postpartum hemorrhage.[88] Similar to plasma, transfusion thresholds for cryoprecipitate remain controversial, although rec-ommended fibrinogen levels range from 100 mg/dL (traditionally indicated for congen-ital hypofibrinogenemia)[23] up to 150 to 200 mg/dL for acquired deficiency secondary to trauma or cardiovascular surgery.[89,90]

In contrast with traditional coagulation markers such as PT-INR, aPTT, and fibrin-ogen, viscoelastic assays in the form of thromboelastography or rotational thromboe-lastometry more closely replicate the process of in vivo clot formation and have the capability of assessing individual components of thrombosis, such as thrombin gen-eration, platelet function, fibrin cross-linking, and fibrinolysis.[91] Given their increasing availability in the clinical setting, these platforms can serve as powerful tools for eval-uating hemostatic potential; individual assay parameters (eg, R time) are already proving useful as therapeutic thresholds to guide transfusion and antifibrinolytic therapy.

SUMMARY

The emergence of new products and therapies is likely to have significant impact on pediatric transfusion therapy because of changing safety profiles in especially vulner-able populations. Pathogen reduction[92] technology has been able to render treated blood products free (or very low risk) of untested or undetected pathogens. This approach to blood product manufacturing holds great promise to decrease the risk of transfusion-transmitted diseases, especially bacterial contamination of platelets. Studies have been done to evaluate the efficacy of the products compared with prod-ucts that are not pathogen reduced. As beneficial as these developments are, a recent pediatric study found that unintended consequences of using such products included lower posttransfusion incremental response and that an increased number of platelet transfusions were needed to maintain certain platelet thresholds.

Current pediatric transfusion practices are informed by a combination of evidence-based recommendations where they exist, expert consensus statements incorpo-rating best practices, guidelines derived from adult populations, and historical prece-dents not supported by data. The persistence of non–evidence-based approaches highlights the ongoing need for additional research targeted toward pediatric populations.

DISCLOSURE

The authors have nothing to disclose.

REFERENCES

1. Hébert PC, Wells G, Blajchman MA, et al. A multicenter, randomized, controlled clinical trial of transfusion requirements in critical care. Transfusion Requirements in Critical Care Investigators, Canadian Critical Care Trials Group. N Engl J Med 1999;340:409–17.
2. Carson JL, Terrin ML, Noveck H, et al. Liberal or restrictive transfusion in high-risk patients after hip surgery. N Engl J Med 2011;365:2453–62.
3. Frey K, editor. Standards for a patient blood management program. 2nd edition. Bethesda (MD): AABB; 2017.
4. Wong ECC, editor. Pediatric transfusion: a physician's handbook. 4th edition. Bethesda (MD): AABB; 2015.
5. Roseff SD, Luban NLC, Manno CS. Guidelines for assessing appropriateness of pediatric transfusion. Transfusion 2002;42:1398–413.
6. Goel R, Cushing M,M, Tobian AAR. Pediatric patient blood management programs: not just transfusing little adults. Transfus Med Rev 2016;30:235–41.
7. Lacroix J, Hébert PC, Hutchison JS, et al. TRI-PICU investigators; Canadian critical care trials group; pediatric acute lung injury and sepsis investigators Network. Transfusion strategies for patients in pediatric intensive care units. N Engl J Med 2007;356(16):1609–19.
8. Lacroix J, Demaret P, Tucci M. Red blood cell transfusion: decision making in pediatric intensive care units. Semin Perinatol 2012;36(4):225–31.
9. Cholette JM, Rubenstein JS, Alfieris GM, et al. Children with single-ventricle physiology do not benefit from higher hemoglobin levels post cavopulmonary connection: results of a prospective, randomized controlled trial of a restrictive versus liberal red-cell transfusion strategy. Pediatr Crit Care Med 2011;12:39–45.
10. Lacritz EM, Hightower AW, Zucker JR, et al. Longitudinal evaluation of severely anemic children in Kenya: the effect of transfusion on mortality and hematologic recovery. AIDS 1997;11:1487–94.
11. Holst LB, Haase N, Wetterslev J, et al. Lower versus higher hemoglobin threshold for transfusion in septic shock. N Engl J Med 2014;371:1381–91.
12. Villanueva C, Colomo A, Bosch A, et al. Transfusion strategies for acute upper gastrointestinal bleeding. N Engl J Med 2013;368:11–21.
13. Jairath V, Kahan BC, Gray A, et al. Restrictive versus liberal blood transfusion for acute upper gastrointestinal bleeding (TRIGGER): a pragmatic, open-label, cluster randomised feasibility trial. Lancet 2015;386:137–44.
14. Robertson CS, Hannay HJ, Yamal J-M, et al. Effect of erythropoietin and transfusion threshold on neurological recovery after traumatic brain injury. JAMA 2014; 312:36–47.
15. Mazer CD, Whitlock RP, Fergusson DA, et al. TRICS investigators and perioperative Anesthesia clinical trials group. Restrictive or liberal red-cell transfusion for cardiac surgery. N Engl J Med 2017;377:2133–44.
16. Mazer CD, Whitlock RP, Fergusson DA, et al. Shehata N; TRICS investigators and perioperative Anesthesia clinical trials group. Six-month outcomes after

restrictive or liberal transfusion for cardiac surgery. N Engl J Med 2018. https://doi.org/10.1056/NEJMoa1808561.

17. de Almeida JP, Vincent J-L, Galas FRBG, et al. Transfusion requirements in surgical oncology patients: a prospective, randomized controlled trial. Anesthesiology 2015;122:29–38.

18. Holst LB, Petersen MW, Haase N, et al. Restrictive versus liberal transfusion strategy for red blood cell transfusion: systematic review of randomized trials with meta-analysis and trial sequential analysis. Br Med J 2015;350:h1354.

19. Carson JL, Stanworth SJ, Roubinian N, et al. Transfusion thresholds and other strategies for guiding allogeneic red blood cell transfusion. Cochrane Database Syst Rev 2016;10:CD002042.

20. Hebert PC, Carson JL. Transfusion threshold of 7 g per deciliter–the new normal. N Engl J Med 2014;371:1459–61.

21. National Institute for Health and Clinical Excellence (NICE). NG 24 blood transfusion. London: NICE; 2015. Available at: www.nice.org.uk/guidance/ng24.

22. Carson JL, Guyatt G, Heddle NM, et al. Clinical practice guidelines from the AABB: red blood cell transfusion thresholds and storage. JAMA 2016;316(19):2025–35.

23. New HV, Berryman J, Bolton-Maggs PHB, et al. Guidelines on transfusion for fetuses, neonates, and older children. Br J Haematol 2016;175:784–828.

24. Gibson BE, Todd A, Roberts I, et al. British Committee for standards in Haematology transfusion Task Force: Writing group: transfusion guidelines for neonates and older children. Br J Haematol 2004;124:433–53.

25. Robitaille N, Lacroix J, Alexandrov L, et al. Excess of veno-occlusive disease in a randomized clinical trial on a higher trigger for red blood cell transfusion after bone marrow transplantation: a Canadian blood and marrow transplant group trial. Biol Blood Marrow Transplant 2013;19:468–73.

26. Tay J, Allan DS, Chatelain E, et al. Liberal versus restrictive red blood cell transfusion thresholds in hematopoietic cell transplantation: a randomized, open label, phase III, noninferiority trial. J Clin Oncol 2020;38:1463–73.

27. Valentine SL, Bembea MM, Muzynski JA, et al. Consensus recommendations for RBC transfusion practice in critically ill children from the pediatric critical care transfusion and anemia expertise initiative. Pediatr Crit Care Med 2018;19(9):884–98.

28. Doctor A, Cholette JM, Remy KE, et al. Recommendations on RBC transfusion in general critically ill children based on hemoglobin and/or physiologic thresholds from the pediatric critical care transfusion and anemia expertise initiative. Pediatr Crit Care Med 2018;19(9):S98–113.

29. Demaret P, Emeriaud G, Hassan NE, et al. Recommendations on RBC transfusions in critically ill children with acute respiratory failure from the pediatric critical care transfusion and anemia expertise initiative. Pediatr Crit Care Med 2018;19(9):S114–20.

30. Muzynski JA, Guzzetta NA, Hall MW, et al. Recommendations on RBC transfusions for critically ill children with nonhemorrhagic shock from the pediatric critical care transfusion and anemia expertise initiative. Pediatr Crit Care Med 2018;19(9):S121–6.

31. Karam O, Russell RT, Stricker P, et al. Recommendations on RBC transfusion in critically ill children with nonlife-threatening bleeding or hemorrhagic shock from the pediatric critical care transfusion and anemia expertise initiative. Pediatr Crit Care Med 2018;19(9):S127–32.

32. Tasker RC, Turgeon AF, Spinella PC, et al. Recommendations on RBC transfusion in critically ill children with acute brain injury from the pediatric critical care transfusion and anemia expertise initiative. Pediatr Crit Care Med 2018;19(9):S133–6.

33. Cholette JM, Willems A, Valentine SL, et al. Recommendations on RBC transfusion in infants and children with acquired and congenital heart disease from the pediatric critical care transfusion and anemia expertise initiative. Pediatr Crit Care Med 2018;19(9):S137–48.

34. Steiner ME, Zantek ND, Stanworth SJ, et al. Recommendations on RBC transfusion support in children with hematologic and oncologic diagnoses from the pediatric critical care transfusion and anemia expertise initiative. Pediatr Crit Care Med 2018;19(9):S149–56.

35. Bembea MM, Cheifetz IM, Fortenberry JD, et al. Recommendations on the indications for RBC transfusion for the critically ill child receiving support from extracorporeal membrane oxygenation, ventricular assist, and renal replacement therapy devices from the pediatric critical care transfusion and anemia expertise initiative. Pediatr Crit Care Med 2018;19(9):S157–62.

36. Zantek ND, Parker RI, van de Watering LM, et al. Recommendations on selection and processing of RBC components for pediatric patients from the pediatric critical care transfusion and anemia expertise initiative. Pediatr Crit Care Med 2018;19(9):S163–9.

37. Patel RM, Josephson C. Neonatal and pediatric platelet transfusions: current concepts and controversies. Curr Opin Hematol 2019;26:466–72.

38. Nellis ME, Karam O, Mauer E, et al. Platelet transfusion practices in critically ill children. Crit Care Med 2018;46:1309–17.

39. Curley A, Stanworth SJ, Willoughby K, et al. Randomized trial of platelet transfusion thresholds in neonates. N Engl J Med 2019;380:242–51.

40. Kumar J, Dutta S, Sundaram V, et al. Platelet transfusion for PDA closure in preterm infants: a randomized controlled trial. Pediatrics 2019;143(5):e20182565.

41. Kaufman RM, Djulbegovic B, Gernsheimer T, et al. Platelet transfusion: a clinical practice guideline from the AABB. Ann Intern Med 2015;162:205–13.

42. Josephson CD, Granger S, Assmann SF, et al. Bleeding risks are higher in children versus adults given prophylactic platelet transfusions for treatment-induced hypoproliferative thrombocytopenia. Blood 2012;120:748–60.

43. Nellis ME, Goel R, Karam O, et al. International study of the epidemiology of platelet transfusions in critically ill children with an underlying oncologic diagnosis. Pediatr Crit Care Med 2019;20:e342–51.

44. Bercovitz RS, Quinones RR. A survey of transfusion practices in pediatric hematopoietic stem cell transplant patients. J Pediatr Hematol Oncol 2013;35:e60–3.

45. Slichter SJ, Kaufman RM, Assmann SF, et al. Dose of prophylactic platelets transfusions and prevention of hemorrhage. N Engl J Med 2010;362:600–13.

46. Bercovitz RS, Josephson CD. Thrombocytopenia and bleeding in pediatric oncology patients. Hematol Am Soc Hematol Educ Program 2012;1:499–505.

47. Kumar A, Mhaskar R, Grossman BJ, et al. Platelet transfusion: a systematic review of the clinical evidence. Transfusion 2015;55:1116–27.

48. Nahirniak S, Slichter SJ, Tanael S, et al. Guidance on platelet transfusion for patients with hypoproliferative thrombocytopenia. Transfus Med Rev 2015;29:3–13.

49. Wandt H, Schaefer-Eckart K, Wendelin K, et al. Therapeutic platelet transfusion versus routine prophylactic transfusion in patients with haematological malignancies: an open-label, multicentre, randomized study. Lancet 2012;380:1309–16.

50. Stanworth SJ, Estcourt LJ, Powter G, et al. A no-prophylaxis platelet-transfusion strategy for hematologic cancers. N Engl J Med 2013;368:1771–80.
51. Stanworth SJ, Estcourt LJ, Llewelyn CA, et al. Impact of prophylactic platelet transfusions on bleeding events in patients with hematologic malignancies: a subgroup analysis of a randomized trial. Transfusion 2014;54:2385–93.
52. Schiffer CA, Bohlke K, Delaney M, et al. Platelet transfusion for patients with cancer: American Society of Clinical Oncology clinical practice guideline update. J Clin Oncol 2018;36:283–99.
53. Estcourt LJ, Malouf R, Hopewell S, et al. Use of platelet transfusions prior to lumbar punctures or epidural anaesthesia for the prevention of complications in people with thrombocytopenia. Cochrane Database Syst Rev 2018;(4):CD011980.
54. Estcourt LJ, Malouf R, Doree C, et al. Prophylactic platelet transfusions prior to surgery for people with a low platelet count. Cochrane Database Syst Rev 2018;(9):CD012779.
55. Howard SC, Gajjar A, Ribeiro RC, et al. Safety of lumbar puncture for children with acute lymphoblastic leukemia and thrombocytopenia. JAMA 2000;284:2222–4.
56. Feusner J. Platelet transfusion "trigger" for lumbar puncture. Pediatr Blood Cancer 2004;43:793.
57. Howard SC, Gajjar AJ, Cheng C, et al. Risk factors for traumatic and bloody lumbar puncture in children with acute lymphoblastic leukemia. JAMA 2002;288:2001–7.
58. Zeidler K, Arn K, Senn O, et al. Optimal preprocedural platelet transfusion threshold for central venous catheter insertions in patients with thrombocytopenia. Transfusion 2011;51:2269–76.
59. Camazine MN, Karam O, Colvin R, et al. Outcomes related to the use of frozen plasma or pooled solvent/detergent-treated plasma in critically ill children. Pediatr Crit Care Med 2017;18:e215–23.
60. Holcomb JB, del Junco DJ, Fox EE, et al. The prospective, observational, multicenter, major trauma transfusion (PROMMTT) study. JAMA Surg 2013;148:127–36.
61. O'Shaughnessy DF, Atterbury C, Bolton Maggs P, et al. Guidelines for the use of fresh-frozen plasma, cryoprecipitate and cryosupernatant. Br J Haematol 2004;126:11–28.
62. Nellis ME, Saini A, Spinella PC, et al. Pediatric plasma and platelet transfusions on extracorporeal membrane oxygenation: a subgroup analysis of two large international point-prevalence studies and the role of local guidelines. Pediatr Crit Care Med 2020;21:267–75.
63. Goldenberg NA, Manco-Johnson MJ. Pediatric hemostasis and use of plasma components. Best Pract Res Clin Haematol 2006;19(1):143–55.
64. Four-factor prothrombin complex concentrate versus plasma for rapid vitamin K antagonist reversal in patients needing urgent surgical or invasive interventions: a phase 3b, open-label, non-inferiority, randomized trial. Lancet 2015;385(9982):2077–87.
65. Milling TJ, Refaai MA, Sarode R, et al. Safety of a four-factor prothrombin complex concentrate versus plasma for vitamin K antagonist reversal: an integrated analysis of two phase IIIb clinical trials. Acad Emerg Med 2016;23(4):466–75.
66. Tinmouth A. Assessing the rationale and effectiveness of frozen plasma transfusions: an evidence-based review. Hematol Oncol Clin North Am 2016;30:561–72.
67. Puetz J, Witmer C, Huan YSV, et al. Widespread use of fresh frozen plasma in US children's hospitals despite limited evidence demonstrating a beneficial effect. J Pediatr 2012;160:210–5.

68. Stanworth SJ, Walsh TS, Prescott RJ, et al. A national study of plasma use in critical care: clinical indications, dose and effect on prothrombin time. Crit Care 2011;15:R108.
69. Soundar EP, Besandre R, Hartman SK, et al. Plasma is ineffective in correcting mildly elevated PT-INR in critically ill children: a retrospective observational study. J Int Care 2014;2:64.
70. Stanworth SJ, Brunskill SJ, Hyde CJ, et al. Is fresh frozen plasma clinically effective? A systematic review of randomized controlled trials. Br J Haematol 2004; 126(1):139–52.
71. Yang L, Stanworth S, Hopewell S, et al. Is fresh frozen plasma clinically effective? An update of a systematic review of randomized controlled trials. Transfusion 2012;52:1673–86.
72. Stanworth SJ, Grant-Casey J, Lowe D, et al. The use of fresh-frozen plasma in England: high levels of inappropriate use in adults and children. Transfusion 2011; 51:62–70.
73. Tinmouth A, Thompson T, Arnold DM, et al. Utilization of frozen plasma in Ontario: a provincewide audit reveals a high rate of inappropriate transfusions. Transfusion 2013;53:2222–9.
74. Lauzier F, Cook D, Griffith L, et al. Fresh frozen plasma transfusion in critically ill patients. Crit Care Med 2007;35(7):1655–9.
75. Karam O, Tucci M, Lacroix J, et al. International survey on plasma transfusion practices in critically ill children. Transfusion 2014;54:1125–32.
76. Karam O, Lacroix J, Robitaille N, et al. Association between plasma transfusions and clinical outcome in critically ill children: a prospective observational study. Vox Sang 2013;104:342–9.
77. Leeper CM, Neal MD, Billiar TR, et al. Overresuscitation with plasma is associated with sustained fibrinolysis shutdown and death in pediatric traumatic brain injury. J Trauma Acute Care Surg 2018;85(1):12–7.
78. Karam O, Demaret P, Shefler a, et al. Indications and effects of plasma transfusions in critically ill children. Am J Respir Crit Care Med 2015;191(12):1395–402.
79. Abdel-Wahab OI, Healy B, Dzik WH. Effect of fresh-frozen plasma transfusion on prothrombin time and bleeding in patients with mild coagulation abnormalities. Transfusion 2006;46:1279–85.
80. Holland LL, Brooks JP. Toward rational fresh frozen plasma transfusion: the effect of plasma transfusion on coagulation test results. Am J Clin Pathol 2006;126: 133–9.
81. Chapin CA, Mohammad S, Bass LM, et al. Liver biopsy can be safely performed in pediatric acute liver failure to aid in diagnosis and management. J Pediatr Gastroenterol Nutr 2018;67(4):441–5.
82. Haas B, Chittams JL, Trerotola SO. Large-bore tunneled central venous catheter insertion in patients with coagulopathy. J Vasc Interv Radiol 2010;21:212–7.
83. Segal JB, Dzik WH. Paucity of studies to support that abnormal coagulation test results predict bleeding in the setting of invasive procedures: an evidence-based review. Transfusion 2005;45:1413–25.
84. Shehata N, Mo YD. Hemotherapy decisions and their outcomes. In: Cohn CS, Delaney M, editors. Technical manual. 20th edition. Bethesda (MD): AABB; 2020.
85. Downey LA, Andrews J, Hedlin H, et al. Fibrinogen concentrate as an alternative to cryoprecipitate in a postcardiopulmonary transfusion algorithm in infants undergoing cardiac surgery: a prospective randomized controlled trial. Anesth Analg 2020;130(3):740–51.

86. Galas FR, de Almeida JP, Fukushima JT, et al. Hemostatic effects of fibrinogen concentrate compared with cryoprecipitate in children after cardiac surgery: a randomized pilot trial. J Thorac Cardiovasc Surg 2014;148(4):1647–55.
87. Callum J, Farkouh ME, Scales DC, et al. Effect of fibrinogen concentrate vs cryoprecipitate on blood component transfusion after cardiac surgery: the FIBRES randomized clinical trial. JAMA 2019;322(20):1–11.
88. Ahmed S, Harrity C, Johnson S, et al. The efficacy of fibrinogen concentrate compared with cryoprecipitate in major obstetric haemorrhage – an observational study. Transfus Med 2012;22:344–9.
89. Levy JH, Goodnough LT. How I use fibrinogen replacement therapy in acquired bleeding. Blood 2015;125(9):1387–93.
90. Karkouti K, Callum J, Crowther MA, et al. The relationship between fibrinogen levels after cardiopulmonary bypass and large volume red cell transfusion in cardiac surgery: an observational study. Anesth Analg 2013;117:14–22.
91. Kane LC, Woodward CS, Husain SA, et al. Thromboelastography – does it impact blood component transfusion in pediatric heart surgery? J Surg Res 2016; 200:21–7.
92. Schulz WL, McPadden L, Gehrie EA, et al. Blood utilization and transfusion reactions in pediatric patients transfused with conventional or pathogen reduced platelets. J Pediatr 2019;209:220–5.

Transfusion in Neonatal Patients
Review of Evidence-Based Guidelines

Patricia E. Zerra, MD[a,b], Cassandra D. Josephson, MD[a,b],*

KEYWORDS

- Transfusion medicine • Neonate • Premature infant • Platelet
- Red blood cell transfusion • Fresh frozen plasma

KEY POINTS

- Transfusion recommendations in neonatal patients are less defined by evidence-based guidelines than those in older children and adults.
- When making the decision to transfuse a neonate, clinicians should consider physiologic differences of this age group, gestational and postnatal age, congenital disorders, and maternal factors.
- Anemia and thrombocytopenia are highly prevalent in preterm neonates, and the risks versus benefits of transfusion must be weighed carefully in this vulnerable population.

INTRODUCTION

Although a critical therapy in the management of hospitalized pediatric patients,[1,2] transfusion of red blood cells (RBCs), platelets, and fresh frozen plasma (FFP) in neonatal patients has not been well characterized in the literature, with few studies describing the indications and recommendations for transfusion in this unique patient population. Anemia and thrombocytopenia are highly prevalent, especially in preterm neonates, with most premature infants in neonatal intensive care units (NICUs) requiring at least 1 transfusion in the first week of life.[3,4]

Physiologic differences between neonates and older infants and children must be taken into account when considering transfusion of blood products. The neonatal period encompasses the first 4 weeks after birth (<28 days old) and includes both full-term (>39 weeks of gestation) as well as premature infants (any neonate born

Funding: This work was supported in part by funding from P01 HL046925 to C. Josephson. Additional funding was from the NICHD Child Health Research Career Development Award Program, K12HD072245, Atlanta Pediatric Scholars Program to P.E. Zerra.
[a] Department of Pathology and Laboratory Medicine, Emory University Hospital, 1364 Clifton Road NE, Atlanta, GA 30322, USA; [b] Aflac Cancer and Blood Disorders Center, Children's Healthcare of Atlanta, Egleston Hospital, 1405 Clifton Rd, Atlanta, GA 30322, USA
* Corresponding author. Whitehead Biomedical Research Building, 615 Michael Street, Room 105M, Atlanta, GA 30322, USA
E-mail address: cjoseph@emory.edu

Clin Lab Med 41 (2021) 15–34
https://doi.org/10.1016/j.cll.2020.10.002
labmed.theclinics.com
0272-2712/21/© 2020 Elsevier Inc. All rights reserved.

before 37 completed weeks of gestation). Most preterm infants requiring transfusion are very low birth weight (VLBW), weighing less than 1500 g, and extremely low birth weight (ELBW), weighing less than 1000 g.[5] When evaluating neonates with anemia, thrombocytopenia, bleeding, or coagulopathy, clinicians should consider gestational and postnatal age, congenital disorders, maternal factors, and transplacental antibody transfer. In addition, neonates have smaller blood volumes relative to larger children or adults, so potentially toxic exposures or antibodies present in transfused products may be more likely to result in clinically relevant consequences.[6,7]

Unlike in the more well-studied adult population, guidelines for transfusion in neonates varies greatly worldwide and between institutions.[8–11] More recently, a growing body of research has focused on delineating neonatal transfusion specifics. This review of the existing literature summarizes current evidence-based neonatal transfusion guidelines and highlights areas of current ongoing research and those in need of future studies.

FETAL AND NEONATAL HEMATOPOIESIS
Term Neonates

When making the decision to transfuse during the neonatal period, it is important to understand fetal and neonatal hematopoiesis. Hemoglobin concentration increases progressively throughout gestation and peaks after birth. Full-term neonates have hemoglobin values of 16 to 17 g/dL at term, which may increase by 1 to 2 g/dL because of placental transfusion at birth and may vary depending on timing of cord clamping. There is a gradual decline in hemoglobin concentration to a nadir of 11 to 12 g/dL at 8 weeks, termed physiologic anemia.[12] Erythropoiesis then accelerates, followed by an increase in hemoglobin level.

Premature Neonates

Physiologic anemia can be more pronounced in premature infants, and the decline in hemoglobin level may occur earlier. In addition, premature infants often have a marked decrease in hemoglobin concentration, termed anemia of prematurity. Anemia of prematurity is caused by a combination of a lower hemoglobin level at birth based on gestational age, reduced RBC lifespan, decreased production of endogenous erythropoietin, hyporegenerative bone marrow, medical complications and frequent blood sampling, all resulting in a limited response to anemia.[13]

NEONATAL RED BLOOD CELL TRANSFUSION

RBC transfusion is a critical intervention to increase oxygen-carrying capacity in anemic neonates. In addition to severe anemia, indications for transfusion in the early neonatal period can include acute blood loss, hypotension, hypovolemia, or to improve oxygen-carrying capacity in infants with respiratory failure.[14] Although often lifesaving, transfusions also have the potential to cause adverse effects, including hemolytic transfusion reactions, alloimmunization, infections, volume overload, allergic reactions, or iron excess.[15,16] Therefore, especially in the vulnerable neonatal population, it is essential to establish guidelines to determine when transfusion is indicated.

Strategies to Limit Red Blood Cell Transfusions in Neonates

Preventive strategies to decrease the incidence of anemia and resultant use of RBC transfusions in neonates have been used, with variable success.

Limiting phlebotomy losses

Phlebotomy-related blood losses can be minimized by alterations in practice, including use of point-of-care devices, minimizing unnecessary laboratory testing, in-line arterial testing, and optimizing frequency and volume of blood draws. In addition, umbilical cord blood can be used for neonatal blood type and screen, complete blood count with differential, and blood culture.[17] Although there is a chance that confirmatory testing may be needed because of interference from Wharton jelly, use of cord blood in initial testing can significantly decrease blood loss caused by phlebotomy. Use of these strategies has been shown to decrease phlebotomy losses and/or the need for RBC transfusion and should be considered, especially in VLBW premature infants.[18]

Delayed cord clamping

Delayed cord clamping ($\geq$30 seconds) has recently been used to increase the initial hematocrit (Hct) of neonates at birth. This practice has been shown to significantly decrease the number of transfusions needed in neonates and is associated with a lower incidence of intraventricular hemorrhage and acute gut injury as well as a decrease in hospital mortality compared with immediate cord clamping.[19–23] However, delayed cord clamping has not been well studied in the group of neonates who most often require transfusion, VLBW neonates. This high-quality evidence supports current guidelines from the American College of Obstetricians and Gynecologists (ACOG) recommending delayed cord clamping in premature infants.[20,22]

Pharmacologic interventions

Recombinant human erythropoietin (EPO) has been used in an attempt to diminish the severity of, or to treat, anemia of prematurity as well as to decrease the need for RBC transfusion in premature neonates. Although EPO has been shown to effectively stimulate erythropoiesis in premature infants, initial studies were conflicting in showing a reduction in the need for RBC transfusion or an improvement in overall neurologic outcome.[24–28] Ohls and colleagues[26] reported that administration of darbepoetin or EPO to premature infants resulted in both a decreased number and volume of transfusions as well as improved cognitive outcome at 18 to 22 months.[27] In contrast, a multicenter randomized controlled trial (PENUT [Preterm Erythropoietin Neuroprotection Trial]) in 2020 found no significant difference in the incidence of death or severe neurodevelopmental impairment at 2 years of age in 741 extremely premature infants that were randomized to receive placebo or high-dose EPO.[28] However, a post hoc analysis reported that infants receiving EPO required transfusion of a significantly decreased volume of RBCs after 10 days of life compared with placebo.[29] Therefore, particularly because patient blood management strategies are critical, EPO is being considered to decrease the need for RBC transfusion in premature infants.

Further contributing to anemia, premature infants have a relative deficiency in iron stores as a result of incomplete iron transport from the mother to the fetus before birth.[30] The use of iron supplementation has been shown to slightly increase the hemoglobin level in premature and low birth weight infants, while improving overall iron stores and decreasing the risk of developing iron deficiency anemia.[31] Of note, a study of VLBW infants showed that both higher cumulative dose of enteral iron supplementation and total volume of RBCs transfused were independently associated with the development of bronchopulmonary dysplasia (BPD).[32] The optimal dosing and timing of iron supplementation as well as mechanisms underlying this association remain to be studied.

Potential Risks of Red Blood Cell Transfusion in Neonates

Determining the optimal hemoglobin concentration at which transfusion is indicated is imperative in premature infants because of their higher likelihood of requiring transfusion resulting from lower hemoglobin levels at birth, iatrogenic losses from phlebotomy, and anemia of prematurity. Although RBC transfusions can be lifesaving for neonates with severe anemia or bleeding, there are inherent risks associated with transfusion that must be considered. In addition, RBC transfusion continues to be studied to determine potential contribution to some of the major causes of morbidity and mortality in preterm infants, including necrotizing enterocolitis (NEC), BPD, intraventricular hemorrhage (IVH), or death.[33–35] In contrast, some studies have raised concerns regarding risks associated with delaying transfusion and allowing more permissive levels of anemia in preterm infants.[36]

Red blood cell transfusion and necrotizing enterocolitis

NEC is a devastating disease in neonates, accounting for 1 in 10 deaths in United States NICUs.[37] The cause of NEC remains incompletely understood and further delineating the underlying risk factors remains an important area of research. Although previous data have been conflicting,[38] a recent study showed that, among VLBW infants, severe anemia ($\leq$8 g/dL) but not RBC transfusion was associated with an increased risk of NEC.[39] In addition, it was also noted that anemic infants were at higher risk of developing NEC than infants with normal hemoglobin concentrations.[36] This finding is further supported by previous studies suggesting that immune dysregulation underlies NEC development,[40–43] combined with recent studies showing an increase in levels of the proinflammatory cytokine interferon gamma in VLBW preterm infants with anemia, suggesting this may predispose them to the development of NEC.[44]

Neurologic outcome in premature neonates

Of particular importance in preterm infants is the development of neuroprotective strategies to improve overall outcome. Large periventricular hemorrhagic infarctions in neonates are associated with poor neurodevelopmental outcomes, and are more likely to occur with wide fluctuations in blood pressure and blood flow through the delicate capillary beds in premature infants.[45] Previous studies have suggested an association between IVH in VLBW infants and transfusions administered during the first few days following delivery.[8,46,47] However, the development of IVH in preterm neonates is certainly multifactorial.[48] Regardless, children born preterm, and especially those that are VLBW, are at higher risk of long-term neurologic sequelae than term infants, including major impairments such as cerebral palsy, intellectual disability, deafness, or blindness,[49,50] as well as behavioral and psychiatric disorders.[51–53] Therefore, it is essential to identify evidence-based transfusion practices in order to define the benefits and risks associated with RBC transfusion, especially in this neurologically vulnerable premature population of infants.

Optimal Red Blood Cell Transfusion Thresholds in Neonates

Two previous large randomized controlled trials (RCTs) designed to define neonatal RBC transfusion thresholds reported conflicting results regarding neurocognitive outcomes in preterm neonates receiving liberal compared with restrictive transfusion thresholds.[54,55] This important issue has been reexamined recently with 2 additional RCTs, with the goal of providing evidence-based recommendations for clinicians (**Table 1**).

Table 1
Multicenter randomized controlled trials comparing liberal versus restrictive red blood cell transfusion in extremely low birth weight infants

Trial	Patient Population	Transfusion Threshold (Hct)	Primary Outcome	Results
ETTNO[56]	1013 premature infants in Europe GA<30 wk; BW<1000 g	Liberal: 28%–41% Restrictive: 21%–34% After randomization, threshold based on postnatal age and health status	Death or neurodevelopmental impairment at 24 mo corrected age	No difference between liberal vs restrictive transfusion; 44.4% vs 42.9%; OR 1.05 (95% CI, 0.80–1.39); $P = .72$
TOP[57]	1824 premature infants in the United States GA 22 to <29 wk; BW<1000g	Liberal: 32%–38% Restrictive: 21%–32% After randomization, threshold based on postnatal age and health status	Survival, neurodevelopmental impairment at 22–26 mo corrected age	Preliminary results with no difference between liberal vs restrictive transfusion

Abbreviations: BW, birth weight; CI, confidence interval; ETTNO, Effect of Transfusion Thresholds on Neurocognitive Outcomes; GA, gestational age; OR, odds ratio; TOP, Transfusion of Prematures .

The Effect of Transfusion Thresholds on Neurocognitive Outcomes trial

Results from the Effect of Transfusion Thresholds on Neurocognitive Outcomes of ELBW infants (ETTNO) trial have recently been published.[56] This RCT, conducted in 36 NICUs in Europe, enrolled ELBW infants who were randomized to receive RBC transfusion based on liberal (Hct 34%–41% in critical and 28%–35% in noncritical infants) versus restrictive (Hct 27%–34% in critical and 21%–28% in noncritical infants) RBC transfusion thresholds. In addition to current state of health, the Hct trigger thresholds of each group were assigned based on postnatal age (<7 days, 8–21 days, or >21 days old). The primary outcome of death or disability (defined as cognitive deficit, cerebral palsy, or severe visual or hearing impairment) at 24 months corrected age did not differ between neonates randomized to liberal or restrictive transfusion groups.

The Transfusion of Prematures trial

The Transfusion of Prematures (TOP) trial is a multicenter study in the United States sponsored by the National Institute of Child Health and Human Development (NCT01702805). It randomizes ELBW infants with gestational age less than 29 weeks to receive RBC transfusion based on a liberal (Hct 32%–38% in infants receiving respiratory support and 29%–35% in infants without respiratory support) or restrictive (Hct 25%–32% in infants receiving respiratory support and 21%–29% in infants without respiratory support) hemoglobin thresholds. Similar to the ETTNO trial, different thresholds were used based on postnatal age. The primary outcome was survival and rates of neurodevelopmental impairment at 22 to 26 months corrected age. Preliminary findings in a recently presented abstract agreed with the findings in the ETTNO trial, showing no difference between infants in the liberal versus restrictive groups.[57]

Limitations to Effect of Transfusion Thresholds on Neurocognitive Outcomes and Transfusion of Prematures trials

The vast heterogeneity of critically ill patients contributes to the difficulty in interpreting the results of clinical trials. An important caveat of both the ETTNO and TOP trials is that neonates were not randomized to the most restrictive Hct levels until they were older than 21 days. Instead, during the first 2 weeks of life, less restrictive thresholds were used. In addition, the restrictive level of ~Hb 8 to 10 g/dL or higher if the infant was critically ill or receiving respiratory support is still higher than the usual restrictive levels used at most institutions for pediatric patients. Thus, although the studies did not observe a difference in primary outcome between the restrictive and liberal transfusion groups, an important question that remains to be determined is whether early anemia and/or prolonged anemia results in potential detrimental effects. Future studies are needed to fully inform clinicians on the proper transfusion support parameters for neonates to achieve the best ultimate outcomes.

Also, of note, the neonatal transfusion trials mentioned earlier function to compare liberal versus restrictive transfusion strategies based on laboratory thresholds alone (hemoglobin or Hct). However, cell count alone may not be an accurate predictor of physiologically relevant outcomes such as tissue oxygen delivery,[58] especially in neonates with varying levels of illness, age, and gestational age. Studies are needed to identify more all-inclusive markers of clinical outcome as well as including long-term outcomes because of the immunomodulatory effects of transfusion that may have effects on neurodevelopment, immunity, and inflammation.

Red Blood Cell Product Selection for Neonates

Once the decision has been made to transfuse RBCs, the most appropriate product must be chosen. There is little guidance available regarding appropriate blood product collection, storage, and pathogen testing in the neonatal population (these topics are covered in more detail in Jenna T. Reece and Deborah Sesok-Pizzini's article, "Inventory Management and Product Selection in Pediatric Blood Banking," in this issue).

Special considerations in neonatal patients include ABO compatibility, total blood volume, immaturity, immunosuppression, immunodeficiencies, and blood donor exposure. Factors to consider when choosing the type of RBC product to administer to a premature infant or neonate include type of anticoagulant-preservative solution (CPDA-1 [citrate phosphate dextrose-adenine 1] vs additive solutions [AS-1, AS-3])[59]; potassium load, which varies depending on the unit storage length; and risk of citrate toxicity. In general, specific RBC product selection recommendations for neonates are not necessary when small-volume transfusions (ie, <20 mL/kg of RBCs) are administered.

Fresh versus stored red blood cells

A recent RCT showed no difference in outcome when using fresh (≤7 days) versus standard-issue RBCs in premature VLBW infants.[60] Accordingly, the clinical practice guidelines from the AABB recommend that standard-issue RBC units are administered to neonates rather than limiting to transfusion of fresh (<10 days) RBC units.[61]

When large-volume transfusions are required, such as in cases of hypotensive shock, extracorporeal membrane oxygenation (ECMO), exchange transfusion, or cardiopulmonary bypass, there is a risk of increases in plasma potassium levels from stored units. In this situation, it may be prudent to consider fresher, washed, or volume-reduced RBCs, which all have lower potassium loads.[62,63] In addition, calcium levels should be closely monitored in neonates requiring multiple transfusions because of the risk of citrate toxicity and resultant hypocalcemia.

ABO group and antibody screen

During pregnancy, transplacental transfer of maternal immunoglobulin G (IgG) antibodies to the fetus can occur, and this can include anti-RBC antibodies. With maternofetal hemorrhage, immunoglobulin M (IgM) antibodies may be transferred. Therefore, when selecting RBC units for transfusion in a neonate, they must be compatible with both the neonatal blood type as well as any maternal antibodies present. Because of this, many institutions transfuse group O RBCs to all neonates; however, ABO-specific blood can be transfused if tests determine there are no anti-A, anti-B, or anti-A,B IgM or IgG maternal antibodies present directed toward the neonate's RBCs.[64]

When performing an antibody screen before transfusion of a neonate, maternal blood can serve as the source because any antibodies present originated in the mother. A negative initial antibody screen in a neonate does not need to be repeated during a hospitalization until 4 months of age,[64] because the immature immune system of a neonate rarely produces antibodies in response to RBC transfusion. If an antibody is detected, antigen-negative units should be provided until it has been determined that the antibody has cleared from the infant's circulation.

Limiting donor exposure

Many institutions attempt to limit donor exposure by reserving specific units for neonates and retrieving sterile docked aliquots for transfusion to be drawn off as needed until outdate of the unit.[5,65,66] Transfusion of aliquots from the same donor in instances where multiple transfusions are required can minimize potential risks that can be associated with transfusion of blood components from multiple donors.

Cytomegalovirus transmission in neonates

Of specific interest in developing neonates is mitigating the risks of transfusion-transmitted (TT) infections with known clinical complications in this vulnerable population. In addition to other groups of immunocompromised patients, premature neonates are a high-risk group for severe disseminated infection from cytomegalovirus (CMV). During latent CMV infection, the virus is associated with mononuclear leukocytes; therefore, leukocyte reduction decreases the risk of TT-CMV.[67–71] A small number of clinical trials have estimated the risk of acquiring CMV from leukocyte-reduced blood to be considerably less than 1%.[67–72] Although small, there remains a risk of asymptomatic CMV-seronegative donors in early stages of infection transmitting CMV through virus particles in plasma.[73,74]

A prospective study of VLBW infants reported no CMV infection after transfusion of 2081 blood products that were both leukocyte reduced and CMV seronegative.[75] Furthermore, a prospective observational study did not find any cases of TT-CMV in VLBW infants who received either leukocyte-reduced blood products or both leukocyte-reduced and CMV-seronegative products.[76] Notably, most neonatal CMV cases result from transmission from the mother, most often by maternal breast milk rather than transfused blood products. Therefore, it is reasonable to assume that leukocyte-reduced blood components reduce the risk of TT-CMV to a level similar to CMV-negative products without window period breakthrough.

In light of the evidence discussed earlier, a reasonable approach is administration of blood products with reduced risk of CMV transmission (CMV seronegative if available or leukocyte reduced) to premature neonates with a birth weight of less than 1500 g before their initial discharge home. Future studies should focus on the efficacy and safety of pathogen-inactivation approaches in neonates, especially for extremely preterm neonates.

NEONATAL PLATELET TRANSFUSION
Thrombocytopenia in Neonates

Thrombocytopenia is common in neonates, and can affect an estimated 1% to 2% of otherwise healthy newborns. Critically ill neonates have an even higher rate of thrombocytopenia, with 20% to 35% having platelets counts of less than 150,000/μL.[77] The incidence increases with decreasing gestational age, with approximately 70% of VLBW neonates experiencing thrombocytopenia.[77,78] The differential diagnosis of thrombocytopenia in neonates is broad, and includes intrauterine infection, placental insufficiency, neonatal sepsis, drugs, and immune thrombocytopenia.[79] Approximately 20% to 25% of affected neonates receive at least 1 platelet transfusion,[78,80] which is administered in most cases not for bleeding but when the platelet count reaches an arbitrary threshold.[10,80]

The incidence of bleeding in neonates increases with decreasing gestational age, with a prospective observational study showing a 63% incidence of bleeding in infants at less than 28 weeks' gestation compared with 14% in infants at greater than 28 weeks' gestation.[81] The most severe bleeding complication in neonates is IVH, which, when present, has the potential to affect long-term neurodevelopmental outcomes.[10] However, the risk of bleeding in neonates does not correlate well with overall platelet counts, making it difficult to determine the proper threshold at which transfusions should be administered.[81]

Physiologic Differences Between Neonatal and Adult Platelets

Platelet function and risk of bleeding are challenging to assess in neonates, because neonatal platelets are hyporeactive to several of the agonists used to test function in the laboratory. Despite this, tests of primary hemostasis are normal or even show shorter bleeding and closure times than in adults.[82,83] In part, this is caused by other differences, including higher Hct and increased von Willebrand factor concentrations in neonates. Ongoing studies focused on the development of tools to evaluate platelet function and whole-blood hemostasis in individual neonates may be able to more specifically address the need for a platelet transfusion.[84] These differences between the neonatal and adult hemostatic systems should be kept in mind when considering transfusion of platelets, and when determining thresholds for transfusion.

Platelet Transfusion Thresholds in the Neonate

The goal of prophylactic platelet transfusion is bleeding prevention; however, neonates' platelet counts and bleeding risks are not directly correlated.[85] Moreover, platelet transfusions have risks.[86] Data are limited to guide platelet transfusion in preterm and more mature neonates, due to limited clinical trials in this patient population.[87] However, 3 recently completed RCTs contribute to improved platelet transfusion strategies in premature neonates (**Table 2**).

A large RCT, performed more than 30 years ago, found there was no increase in the development of new intracranial hemorrhage (ICH) or worsening of existing ICH when premature thrombocytopenic infants were randomized to receive platelet transfusions at thresholds of either 50,000 or 150,000/μL. The study did conclude that there was a decreased use of FFP and RBC transfusions when transfusing platelets at a higher threshold.[88] However, the lower threshold in the study (50,000/μL) is significantly higher than that used commonly in current clinical practice.

Most recently, in 2019, the Platelet Transfusion Thresholds in Premature Neonates (PlaNeT-2) RCT compared 2 different platelet transfusion thresholds (25,000/μL vs 50,000/μL) in premature infants born at a gestational age less than 34 weeks.[89] They reported a significantly higher incidence of death or major bleeding in the group of neonates receiving platelet transfusion with a threshold of 50,000/μL compared with those randomized to receive transfusion at a threshold of 25,000/μL. Moreover, there was also a higher incidence of BPD in the higher threshold group, further supporting the use of a more restrictive transfusion threshold in premature infants.

A subanalysis of the PlaNeT-2 trial more closely examined the risk of major bleeding or death in the lowest-risk and highest-risk infants included in the trial. Regardless of risk category, neonates had a better outcome when a lower platelet count threshold was used, with the highest-risk infants gaining the greatest benefit.[86] Additional studies have provided further evidence to support lower platelet transfusion thresholds in nonbleeding premature neonates.[85,90,91]

A third recent RCT reported that there was no effect of platelet transfusion threshold (100,000/μL vs 20,000/μL) on time to closure of patent ductus arteriosus (PDA) in premature neonates.[92] However, the investigators did note more cases of IVH among the infants receiving platelet transfusions to keep platelet count greater than 100,000/μL.

Limitations of previous platelet threshold trials

These studies support the implementation of a restrictive platelet transfusion guideline in premature infants. However, premature neonates included in these studies were of a wide range of postnatal and gestational ages. In addition, the clinical status of the neonate should be considered in order to determine the proper platelet threshold. A study investigating full-term neonates is needed, as is one examining VLBW

Table 2
Randomized controlled trials comparing liberal versus restricted platelet transfusion in extremely low birth weight infants

Trial	Patient Population	Platelet Thresholds	Primary Outcome	Results
Andrew et al,[88] 1993	152 infants GA<33 wk; BW, 500–1500 g; platelet count <150,000/μL during the first 72 h of life	150,000/μL vs 50,000/μL	Incidence or extension of ICH	No difference in new/worsening ICH between higher and lower threshold (28% vs 26%, P = .73); higher threshold received less FFP and RBCs
Curley et al,[89] 2019 PlaNeT-2 Trial	660 infants GA<34 wk; platelet count <50,000/μL	50,000/μL vs 25,000/μL	Death or new major bleeding	Higher rates of death or major bleeding in higher threshold group OR, 1.57; 95% CI, 1.06–2.32; P = .02
Kumar et al,[92] 2019	44 infants GA<35 wk; PDA detected at <14 d of age; platelet count <100,000/μL	100,000/μL vs 20,000/μL	Mean time to PDA closure	No significant difference in time to PDA closure; adjusted HR 1.4 (95% CI, 0.57–3.47), P = .46

Abbreviations: HR, hazard ratio; ICH, intracranial hemorrhage; PDA, patent ductus arteriosus; PlaNet-2, Platelet Transfusion Thresholds in Premature Neonates.

premature infants and the most critically ill neonates to more clearly define the effect of lower thresholds during the first week of life and the highest-risk period of bleeding.[93]

Current neonatal platelet transfusion recommendations

With the currently available studies, a reasonable approach for VLBW infants is to transfuse for platelet levels less than 25,000/μL if not bleeding, more than 7 day old, and not having a procedure in the next 24 hours. For other groups of neonates, the platelet transfusion threshold should take into account the patient's clinical severity and risk of bleeding, as well as risk of other comorbidities that may be associated with platelet transfusion. In general, platelet transfusions are indicated when there is significant thrombocytopenia with active bleeding, or when there is an increased risk of IVH, which is typically defined as a platelet count of less than 30,000/μL.

Platelet Product Selection in Neonates

This article briefly discusses the issue of ABO-mismatched platelet transfusions in the neonatal population (product selection is covered in great detail in Jenna T. Reece and Deborah Sesok-Pizzini's article, "Inventory Management and Product Selection in Pediatric Blood Banking," in this issue). ABO-compatible or ABO-identical platelets are ideally transfused to avoid the transfer of incompatible isohemagglutinins (anti-A, anti-B, or anti-A,B antibodies) found in plasma to the recipients, resulting in potential RBC hemolysis.[7,94] Although uncommon, there are case reports describing morbidity and mortality in neonates and children receiving ABO-incompatible platelet transfusions.[7,95–97] In most cases, O-donor platelets (containing anti-A) have resulted in complications in patients with blood type A. This possibility is of particular concern in neonates, particularly premature and VLBW infants, because of their small plasma volumes and inability to dilute out the passive transfer of antibodies following platelet transfusion. Therefore, all attempts should be made to administer ABO-identical or ABO-compatible platelet transfusion in this population. However, because it can be difficult to obtain ABO-compatible platelets because of product shortages, alternative, although not ideal, strategies include washing or volume reducing ABO-mismatched platelets. In addition, although further research is needed to determine ideal safe antithetical antibody titers, administration of low-titer anti-A platelet units to neonates in these situations would be reasonable.[7]

Fetal and Neonatal Alloimmune Thrombocytopenia

Fetal and neonatal alloimmune thrombocytopenia (FNAIT) is the result of passively acquired maternal IgG antiplatelet antibodies that cross the placenta and mediate destruction of fetal platelets. Most cases of FNAIT are the result of maternal antibodies developing against the paternally inherited platelet antigen human platelet antigen 1a (HPA-1a), but it can also include several other antigens, with their incidence depending on the mother's ancestry.[98–101]

FNAIT occurs in 1 to 10 per 10,000 live births, with severe thrombocytopenia and ICH occurring in 3 to 10 per 100,000 infants.[102–104] Roughly 40% to 60% of cases of FNAIT affect a woman's first pregnancy, and ~90% of subsequent pregnancies are affected, with severe disease occurring more often. Severely affected infants have early-onset severe thrombocytopenia and bleeding, including petechiae, purpura, and mucocutaneous bleeding. There is a 10% to 20% risk of neonates with platelet counts of less than 50,000/μL developing ICH.[99]

Although maternal antibodies are cleared within 1 to 3 weeks, because of the risk of severe bleeding during this time, treatment may be indicated. There is variable evidence of the efficacy of intravenous immunoglobulin and corticosteroids in increasing the platelet count in neonates affected by neonatal alloimmune thrombocytopenia (NAIT).[105,106] Platelet transfusion may be indicated prophylactically in the first week of life for platelet counts less than 50,000/μL, with a more restrictive threshold of 30,000/μL often used in stable infants afterward. Bleeding infants with thrombocytopenia and suspected NAIT should receive transfusion of the most readily available platelet unit without delay. Use of platelets that express the targeted antigen transiently increase the platelet count, although transfusion of antigen-negative platelets or washed and irradiated maternal platelets may be needed.[107-110]

NEONATAL PLASMA TRANSFUSION

Plasma transfusion in neonates is often used incorrectly.[111-116] In part, this may be because of the lack of evidence-based guidelines available to guide transfusion of FFP in the pediatric patient population. It is essential to determine the clinical scenarios in neonates that require transfusion of plasma and to differentiate those in which an alternative product, such as a specific factor concentrate, should be used. Of note, in the absence of bleeding, plasma should not be transfused empirically, or for an increased International Normalized Ratio alone.[112-118] In addition, plasma is not indicated for volume expansion, and routine and prophylactic use of plasma has not been shown to reduce the mortality of premature infants.[119]

Indications for Plasma Transfusion

Although evidence-based guidelines are scarce in the neonatal population, there are several clinical conditions in neonates that require the transfusion of plasma. Sepsis, disseminated intravascular coagulopathy, liver disease, congenital or acquired vitamin K deficiency, trauma, and dilutional effects of massive transfusion all have the potential to result in global coagulopathy in neonates.[120-124]

In patients diagnosed with suspected or confirmed congenital thrombotic thrombocytopenic purpura, therapeutic plasma exchange should be performed with plasma as the replacement fluid to replenish ADAMTS13 (a disintegrin and metalloproteinase with a thrombospondin type 1 motif, member 13).[125] Plasma is also used to reconstitute whole blood to be used for neonatal exchange transfusion as well as, in some cases, to prime both cardiothoracic surgery circuits and ECMO circuits. However, there is variability between institutions and conflicting data on the best combination of products to use when priming circuits.[126-131]

Coagulation factor deficiencies

It can be difficult to establish a diagnosis of a specific coagulation factor deficiency caused by physiologically decreased levels of some coagulation proteins in neonates as a result of the normal development of the coagulation system. For example, most coagulation factors in a neonate (factors II, VII, IX and X, XI and XII) are at roughly 50% of the adult levels and gradually increase until 6 months of age. In contrast, levels of factors V and XIII and fibrinogen at birth are similar to adult levels, and factor VIII and von Willebrand factor levels increase at birth and remain increased for the first 6 months.[132] This functional immaturity of the coagulation system can lead to challenges interpreting results and reaching a diagnosis.

Plasma is indicated to replace specific coagulation factors when factor concentrates are not available, particularly factors V and XI, for which specific factor concentrates are not available in the United States.[117,118,133,134] In addition, if a congenital bleeding disorder is suspected, it is prudent to administer plasma in bleeding patients while awaiting definitive testing.[122]

DISCLOSURE

The authors have nothing to disclose.

REFERENCES

1. Jacquot C, Mo YD, Luban NLC. New approaches and trials in pediatric transfusion medicine. Hematol Oncol Clin North Am 2019;33(3):507–20.
2. Cure P, Bembea M, Chou S, et al. 2016 proceedings of the National Heart, Lung, and Blood Institute's scientific priorities in pediatric transfusion medicine. Transfusion 2017;57(6):1568–81.
3. Levy GJ, Strauss RG, Hume H, et al. National survey of neonatal transfusion practices: I. Red blood cell therapy. Pediatrics 1993;91(3):523–9.
4. Hume H, Blanchette V, Strauss RG, et al. A survey of Canadian neonatal blood transfusion practices. Transfus Sci 1997;18(1):71–80.
5. Fabres J, Wehrli G, Marques MB, et al. Estimating blood needs for very-low-birth-weight infants. Transfusion 2006;46(11):1915–20.
6. Zubairi H, Visintainer P, Fleming J, et al. Lead exposure in preterm infants receiving red blood cell transfusions. Pediatr Res 2015;77(6):814–8.
7. Josephson CD, Castillejo MI, Grima K, et al. ABO-mismatched platelet transfusions: strategies to mitigate patient exposure to naturally occurring hemolytic antibodies. Transfus Apher Sci 2010;42(1):83–8.
8. Bednarek FJ, Weisberger S, Richardson DK, et al. Variations in blood transfusions among newborn intensive care units. SNAP II Study Group. J Pediatr 1998;133(5):601–7.
9. Kahn DJ, Richardson DK, Billett HH. Inter-NICU variation in rates and management of thrombocytopenia among very low birth-weight infants. J Perinatol 2003; 23(4):312–6.
10. Josephson CD, Su LL, Christensen RD, et al. Platelet transfusion practices among neonatologists in the United States and Canada: results of a survey. Pediatrics 2009;123(1):278–85.
11. Cremer M, Sola-Visner M, Roll S, et al. Platelet transfusions in neonates: practices in the United States vary significantly from those in Austria, Germany, and Switzerland. Transfusion 2011;51(12):2634–41.
12. Orkin SH, Nathan DG. Nathan and Oski's hematology of infancy and childhood. 7th edition. Philadelphia: Saunders/Elsevier; 2009.
13. Doyle JJ. The role of erythropoietin in the anemia of prematurity. Semin Perinatol 1997;21(1):20–7.
14. Roseff SD, Luban NL, Manno CS. Guidelines for assessing appropriateness of pediatric transfusion. Transfusion 2002;42(11):1398–413.
15. Oakley FD, Woods M, Arnold S, et al. Transfusion reactions in pediatric compared with adult patients: a look at rate, reaction type, and associated products. Transfusion 2015;55(3):563–70.
16. Vossoughi S, Perez G, Whitaker BI, et al. Analysis of pediatric adverse reactions to transfusions. Transfusion 2018;58(1):60–9.
17. Carroll PD, Livingston E, Baer VL, et al. Evaluating otherwise-discarded umbilical cord blood as a source for a Neonate's complete blood cell count at various time points. Neonatology 2018;114(1):82–6.
18. Christensen RD, Carroll PD, Josephson CD. Evidence-based advances in transfusion practice in neonatal intensive care units. Neonatology 2014;106(3): 245–53.

19. Rabe H, Gyte GM, Diaz-Rossello JL, et al. Effect of timing of umbilical cord clamping and other strategies to influence placental transfusion at preterm birth on maternal and infant outcomes. Cochrane Database Syst Rev 2019;(9):CD003248.

20. Committee on Obstetric Practice. Committee opinion no. 684: delayed umbilical cord clamping after birth. Obstet Gynecol 2017;129(1):e5–10.

21. Andersson O, Domellof M, Andersson D, et al. Effect of delayed vs early umbilical cord clamping on iron status and neurodevelopment at age 12 months: a randomized clinical trial. JAMA Pediatr 2014;168(6):547–54.

22. Leslie MS, Greene J, Schulkin J, et al. Umbilical cord clamping practices of U.S. obstetricians. J Neonatal Perinatal Med 2018;11(1):51–60.

23. Fogarty M, Osborn DA, Askie L, et al. Delayed vs early umbilical cord clamping for preterm infants: a systematic review and meta-analysis. Am J Obstet Gynecol 2018;218(1):1–18.

24. Donato H, Vain N, Rendo P, et al. Effect of early versus late administration of human recombinant erythropoietin on transfusion requirements in premature infants: results of a randomized, placebo-controlled, multicenter trial. Pediatrics 2000;105(5):1066–72.

25. Maier RF, Obladen M, Muller-Hansen I, et al. Early treatment with erythropoietin beta ameliorates anemia and reduces transfusion requirements in infants with birth weights below 1000 g. J Pediatr 2002;141(1):8–15.

26. Ohls RK, Christensen RD, Kamath-Rayne BD, et al. A randomized, masked, placebo-controlled study of darbepoetin alfa in preterm infants. Pediatrics 2013;132(1):e119–27.

27. Ohls RK, Kamath-Rayne BD, Christensen RD, et al. Cognitive outcomes of preterm infants randomized to darbepoetin, erythropoietin, or placebo. Pediatrics 2014;133(6):1023–30.

28. Juul SE, Comstock BA, Wadhawan R, et al. A randomized trial of erythropoietin for neuroprotection in preterm infants. N Engl J Med 2020;382(3):233–43.

29. Juul SE, Vu PT, Comstock BA, et al. Effect of high-dose erythropoietin on blood transfusions in extremely low gestational age neonates: post hoc analysis of a randomized clinical trial. JAMA Pediatr 2020;174(10):933–43.

30. Aher S, Malwatkar K, Kadam S. Neonatal anemia. Semin Fetal Neonatal Med 2008;13(4):239–47.

31. Mills RJ, Davies MW. Enteral iron supplementation in preterm and low birth weight infants. Cochrane Database Syst Rev 2012;(3):CD005095.

32. Patel RM, Knezevic A, Yang J, et al. Enteral iron supplementation, red blood cell transfusion, and risk of bronchopulmonary dysplasia in very-low-birth-weight infants. Transfusion 2019;59(5):1675–82.

33. Ghirardello S, Dusi E, Cortinovis I, et al. Effects of red blood cell transfusions on the risk of developing complications or death: an observational study of a cohort of very low birth weight infants. Am J Perinatol 2017;34(1):88–95.

34. Wang YC, Chan OW, Chiang MC, et al. Red blood cell transfusion and clinical outcomes in extremely low birth weight preterm infants. Pediatr Neonatol 2017;58(3):216–22.

35. Keir A, Pal S, Trivella M, et al. Adverse effects of red blood cell transfusions in neonates: a systematic review and meta-analysis. Transfusion 2016;56(11):2773–80.

36. Le VT, Klebanoff MA, Talavera MM, et al. Transient effects of transfusion and feeding advances (volumetric and caloric) on necrotizing enterocolitis development: a case-crossover study. PLoS One 2017;12(6):e0179724.

37. Jacob J, Kamitsuka M, Clark RH, et al. Etiologies of NICU deaths. Pediatrics 2015;135(1):e59–65.
38. Mohamed A, Shah PS. Transfusion associated necrotizing enterocolitis: a meta-analysis of observational data. Pediatrics 2012;129(3):529–40.
39. Patel RM, Knezevic A, Shenvi N, et al. Association of red blood cell transfusion, anemia, and necrotizing enterocolitis in very low-birth-weight infants. JAMA 2016;315(9):889–97.
40. Liu Z, Sun X, Tang J, et al. Intestinal inflammation and tissue injury in response to heat stress and cooling treatment in mice. Mol Med Rep 2011;4(3):437–43.
41. De Plaen IG. Inflammatory signaling in necrotizing enterocolitis. Clin Perinatol 2013;40(1):109–24.
42. Hunter CJ, De Plaen IG. Inflammatory signaling in NEC: role of NF-kappaB, cytokines and other inflammatory mediators. Pathophysiology 2014;21(1):55–65.
43. Maheshwari A, Schelonka RL, Dimmitt RA, et al. Cytokines associated with necrotizing enterocolitis in extremely-low-birth-weight infants. Pediatr Res 2014;76(1):100–8.
44. Arthur CM, Nalbant D, Feldman HA, et al. Anemia induces gut inflammation and injury in an animal model of preterm infants. Transfusion 2019;59(4):1233–45.
45. Bassan H. Intracranial hemorrhage in the preterm infant: understanding it, preventing it. Clin Perinatol 2009;36(4):737–62, v.
46. Baer VL, Lambert DK, Henry E, et al. Among very-low-birth-weight neonates is red blood cell transfusion an independent risk factor for subsequently developing a severe intraventricular hemorrhage? Transfusion 2011;51(6):1170–8.
47. Baer VL, Lambert DK, Henry E, et al. Red blood cell transfusion of preterm neonates with a Grade 1 intraventricular hemorrhage is associated with extension to a Grade 3 or 4 hemorrhage. Transfusion 2011;51(9):1933–9.
48. Ballabh P. Intraventricular hemorrhage in premature infants: mechanism of disease. Pediatr Res 2010;67(1):1–8.
49. Sharp M, French N, McMichael J, et al. Survival and neurodevelopmental outcomes in extremely preterm infants 22-24 weeks of gestation born in Western Australia. J Paediatr Child Health 2018;54(2):188–93.
50. Jarjour IT. Neurodevelopmental outcome after extreme prematurity: a review of the literature. Pediatr Neurol 2015;52(2):143–52.
51. Franz AP, Bolat GU, Bolat H, et al. Attention-deficit/hyperactivity disorder and very preterm/very low birth weight: a meta-analysis. Pediatrics 2018;141(1).
52. Joseph RM, O'Shea TM, Allred EN, et al. Prevalence and associated features of autism spectrum disorder in extremely low gestational age newborns at age 10 years. Autism Res 2017;10(2):224–32.
53. Treyvaud K, Ure A, Doyle LW, et al. Psychiatric outcomes at age seven for very preterm children: rates and predictors. J Child Psychol Psychiatry 2013;54(7):772–9.
54. Kirpalani H, Whyte RK, Andersen C, et al. The Premature Infants in Need of Transfusion (PINT) study: a randomized, controlled trial of a restrictive (low) versus liberal (high) transfusion threshold for extremely low birth weight infants. J Pediatr 2006;149(3):301–7.
55. Bell EF, Strauss RG, Widness JA, et al. Randomized trial of liberal versus restrictive guidelines for red blood cell transfusion in preterm infants. Pediatrics 2005;115(6):1685–91.
56. Franz AR, Engel C, Bassler D, et al. Effects of liberal vs restrictive transfusion thresholds on survival and neurocognitive outcomes in extremely low-birth-weight infants: the ETTNO randomized clinical trial. JAMA 2020;324(6):560–70.

57. Kirpalani H, Bell EF, Johnson KJ, et al. A randomized trial of higher versus lower hemoglobin thresholds for extremely low birth weight (ELBW) infants: the Transfusion of Prematures (TOP) Trial. 2020. Available at: https://plan.core-apps.com/pas2020/abstract/6edec56c63f592adb37f205ea944d7d8. Accessed 29 October, 2020.

58. Mintzer JP, Parvez B, Chelala M, et al. Monitoring regional tissue oxygen extraction in neonates <1250 g helps identify transfusion thresholds independent of hematocrit. J Neonatal Perinatal Med 2014;7(2):89–100.

59. Luban NL, Strauss RG, Hume HA. Commentary on the safety of red cells preserved in extended-storage media for neonatal transfusions. Transfusion 1991;31(3):229–35.

60. Fergusson DA, Hebert P, Hogan DL, et al. Effect of fresh red blood cell transfusions on clinical outcomes in premature, very low-birth-weight infants: the ARIPI randomized trial. JAMA 2012;308(14):1443–51.

61. Carson JL, Guyatt G, Heddle NM, et al. Clinical practice guidelines from the AABB: red blood cell transfusion thresholds and storage. JAMA 2016;316(19):2025–35.

62. Sesok-Pizzini D, Pizzini MA. Hyperkalemic cardiac arrest in pediatric patients undergoing massive transfusion: unplanned emergencies. Transfusion 2014;54(1):4–7.

63. Lee AC, Reduque LL, Luban NL, et al. Transfusion-associated hyperkalemic cardiac arrest in pediatric patients receiving massive transfusion. Transfusion 2014;54(1):244–54.

64. Cohn C, Delaney M, Johnson S, et al. Technical manual. 20th edition. Bethesda (MD): AABB; 2020.

65. Cook S, Gunter J, Wissel M. Effective use of a strategy using assigned red cell units to limit donor exposure for neonatal patients. Transfusion 1993;33(5):379–83.

66. Wang-Rodriguez J, Mannino FL, Liu E, et al. A novel strategy to limit blood donor exposure and blood waste in multiply transfused premature infants. Transfusion 1996;36(1):64–70.

67. Strauss RG. Leukocyte-reduction to prevent transfusion-transmitted cytomegalovirus infections. Pediatr Transplant 1999;3(Suppl 1):19–22.

68. Vamvakas EC. Is white blood cell reduction equivalent to antibody screening in preventing transmission of cytomegalovirus by transfusion? A review of the literature and meta-analysis. Transfus Med Rev 2005;19(3):181–99.

69. Kekre N, Tokessy M, Mallick R, et al. Is cytomegalovirus testing of blood products still needed for hematopoietic stem cell transplant recipients in the era of universal leukoreduction? Biol Blood Marrow Transplant 2013;19(12):1719–24.

70. Nash T, Hoffmann S, Butch S, et al. Safety of leukoreduced, cytomegalovirus (CMV)-untested components in CMV-negative allogeneic human progenitor cell transplant recipients. Transfusion 2012;52(10):2270–2.

71. Thiele T, Kruger W, Zimmermann K, et al. Transmission of cytomegalovirus (CMV) infection by leukoreduced blood products not tested for CMV antibodies: a single-center prospective study in high-risk patients undergoing allogeneic hematopoietic stem cell transplantation (CME). Transfusion 2011;51(12):2620–6.

72. Strauss RG. Data-driven blood banking practices for neonatal RBC transfusions. Transfusion 2000;40(12):1528–40.

73. Ziemann M, Krueger S, Maier AB, et al. High prevalence of cytomegalovirus DNA in plasma samples of blood donors in connection with seroconversion. Transfusion 2007;47(11):1972–83.

74. Ziemann M, Heuft HG, Frank K, et al. Window period donations during primary cytomegalovirus infection and risk of transfusion-transmitted infections. Transfusion 2013;53(5):1088–94.

75. Josephson CD, Caliendo AM, Easley KA, et al. Blood transfusion and breast milk transmission of cytomegalovirus in very low-birth-weight infants: a prospective cohort study. JAMA Pediatr 2014;168(11):1054–62.

76. Delaney M, Mayock D, Knezevic A, et al. Postnatal cytomegalovirus infection: a pilot comparative effectiveness study of transfusion safety using leukoreduced-only transfusion strategy. Transfusion 2016;56(8):1945–50.

77. Castle V, Andrew M, Kelton J, et al. Frequency and mechanism of neonatal thrombocytopenia. J Pediatr 1986;108(5 Pt 1):749–55.

78. Christensen RD, Henry E, Wiedmeier SE, et al. Thrombocytopenia among extremely low birth weight neonates: data from a multihospital healthcare system. J Perinatol 2006;26(6):348–53.

79. Roberts IA, Murray NA. Thrombocytopenia in the newborn. Curr Opin Pediatr 2003;15(1):17–23.

80. Dohner ML, Wiedmeier SE, Stoddard RA, et al. Very high users of platelet transfusions in the neonatal intensive care unit. Transfusion 2009;49(5):869–72.

81. Stanworth SJ, Clarke P, Watts T, et al. Prospective, observational study of outcomes in neonates with severe thrombocytopenia. Pediatrics 2009;124(5):e826–34.

82. Andrew M, Paes B, Bowker J, et al. Evaluation of an automated bleeding time device in the newborn. Am J Hematol 1990;35(4):275–7.

83. Israels SJ, Cheang T, McMillan-Ward EM, et al. Evaluation of primary hemostasis in neonates with a new in vitro platelet function analyzer. J Pediatr 2001;138(1):116–9.

84. Deschmann E, Sola-Visner M, Saxonhouse MA. Primary hemostasis in neonates with thrombocytopenia. J Pediatr 2014;164(1):167–72.

85. Muthukumar P, Venkatesh V, Curley A, et al. Severe thrombocytopenia and patterns of bleeding in neonates: results from a prospective observational study and implications for use of platelet transfusions. Transfus Med 2012;22(5):338–43.

86. Fustolo-Gunnink SF, Fijnvandraat K, van Klaveren D, et al. Preterm neonates benefit from low prophylactic platelet transfusion threshold despite varying risk of bleeding or death. Blood 2019;134(26):2354–60.

87. Patel RM, Josephson C. Neonatal and pediatric platelet transfusions: current concepts and controversies. Curr Opin Hematol 2019;26(6):466–72.

88. Andrew M, Vegh P, Caco C, et al. A randomized, controlled trial of platelet transfusions in thrombocytopenic premature infants. J Pediatr 1993;123(2):285–91.

89. Curley A, Stanworth SJ, Willoughby K, et al. Randomized trial of platelet-transfusion thresholds in neonates. N Engl J Med 2019;380(3):242–51.

90. Patel RM, Josephson CD, Shenvi N, et al. Platelet transfusions and mortality in necrotizing enterocolitis. Transfusion 2019;59(3):981–8.

91. Ferrer-Marin F, Chavda C, Lampa M, et al. Effects of in vitro adult platelet transfusions on neonatal hemostasis. J Thromb Haemost 2011;9(5):1020–8.

92. Kumar J, Dutta S, Sundaram V, et al. Platelet transfusion for PDA closure in preterm infants: a randomized controlled trial. Pediatrics 2019;143(5).

93. Sola-Visner MC. Platelet transfusions in neonates - less is more. N Engl J Med 2019;380(3):287–8.

94. Harris SB, Josephson CD, Kost CB, et al. Nonfatal intravascular hemolysis in a pediatric patient after transfusion of a platelet unit with high-titer anti-A. Transfusion 2007;47(8):1412–7.

95. Conway LT, Scott EP. Acute hemolytic transfusion reaction due to ABO incompatible plasma in a plateletapheresis concentrate. Transfusion 1984;24(5): 413–4.

96. Valbonesi M, De Luigi MC, Lercari G, et al. Acute intravascular hemolysis in two patients transfused with dry-platelet units obtained from the same ABO incompatible donor. Int J Artif Organs 2000;23(9):642–6.

97. Angiolillo A, Luban NL. Hemolysis following an out-of-group platelet transfusion in an 8-month-old with Langerhans cell histiocytosis. J Pediatr hematology/oncology 2004;26(4):267–9.

98. Davoren A, Curtis BR, Aster RH, et al. Human platelet antigen-specific alloantibodies implicated in 1162 cases of neonatal alloimmune thrombocytopenia. Transfusion 2004;44(8):1220–5.

99. Ghevaert C, Campbell K, Walton J, et al. Management and outcome of 200 cases of fetomaternal alloimmune thrombocytopenia. Transfusion 2007;47(5): 901–10.

100. Rousseau J, Goldman M, David M. HPA-5b (Bra) neonatal alloimmune thrombocytopenia in Quebec: incidence and clinical outcome in 31 cases. Transfusion 2004;44(6):844–8.

101. Schmidt AE, Sahai T, Refaai MA, et al. Severe platelet transfusion refractoriness in association with antibodies against CD36. Lab Med 2020;51(5):540–4.

102. Burrows RF, Kelton JG. Fetal thrombocytopenia and its relation to maternal thrombocytopenia. N Engl J Med 1993;329(20):1463–6.

103. Knight M, Pierce M, Allen D, et al. The incidence and outcomes of fetomaternal alloimmune thrombocytopenia: a UK national study using three data sources. Br J Haematol 2011;152(4):460–8.

104. Kamphuis MM, Paridaans NP, Porcelijn L, et al. Incidence and consequences of neonatal alloimmune thrombocytopenia: a systematic review. Pediatrics 2014; 133(4):715–21.

105. Calhoun DA, Christensen RD, Edstrom CS, et al. Consistent approaches to procedures and practices in neonatal hematology. Clin Perinatol 2000;27(3): 733–53.

106. Althaus J, Blakemore KJ. Fetomaternal alloimmune thrombocytopenia: the questions that still remain. J Matern Fetal Neonatal Med 2007;20(9):633–7.

107. Bakchoul T, Bassler D, Heckmann M, et al. Management of infants born with severe neonatal alloimmune thrombocytopenia: the role of platelet transfusions and intravenous immunoglobulin. Transfusion 2014;54(3):640–5.

108. Kiefel V, Bassler D, Kroll H, et al. Antigen-positive platelet transfusion in neonatal alloimmune thrombocytopenia (NAIT). Blood 2006;107(9):3761–3.

109. Peterson JA, McFarland JG, Curtis BR, et al. Neonatal alloimmune thrombocytopenia: pathogenesis, diagnosis and management. Br J Haematol 2013; 161(1):3–14.

110. Blanchette VS, Johnson J, Rand M. The management of alloimmune neonatal thrombocytopenia. Best Practice and Research: Clinical Haematology 2000; 13(3):365–90.

111. Puetz J, Witmer C, Huang YS, et al. Widespread use of fresh frozen plasma in US children's hospitals despite limited evidence demonstrating a beneficial effect. J Pediatr 2012;160(2):210–5.e1.
112. Motta M, Del Vecchio A, Perrone B, et al. Fresh frozen plasma use in the NICU: a prospective, observational, multicentred study. Arch Dis Child Fetal Neonatal Ed 2014;99(4):F303–8.
113. Stanworth SJ, Grant Casey J, Lowe D, et al. The use of fresh-frozen plasma in England: high levels of inappropriate use in adults and children. Transfusion 2011;51(1):62–70.
114. Karam O, Tucci M, Lacroix J, et al. International survey on plasma transfusion practices in critically ill children. Transfusion 2014;54(4):1125–32.
115. Poterjoy BS, Josephson CD. Platelets, frozen plasma, and cryoprecipitate: what is the clinical evidence for their use in the neonatal intensive care unit? Semin Perinatol 2009;33(1):66–74.
116. Karam O, Demaret P, Shefler A, et al. Indications and effects of plasma transfusions in critically ill children. Am J Respir Crit Care Med 2015;191(12):1395–402.
117. O'Shaughnessy DF, Atterbury C, Bolton Maggs P, et al. Guidelines for the use of fresh-frozen plasma, cryoprecipitate and cryosupernatant. Br J Haematol 2004; 126(1):11–28.
118. Goldenberg NA, Manco-Johnson MJ. Pediatric hemostasis and use of plasma components. Best Pract Res Clin Haematol 2006;19(1):143–55.
119. A randomized trial comparing the effect of prophylactic intravenous fresh frozen plasma, gelatin or glucose on early mortality and morbidity in preterm babies. The Northern Neonatal Nursing Initiative [NNNI] Trial Group. Eur J Pediatr 1996;155(7):580–8.
120. Maw G, Furyk C. Pediatric massive transfusion: a systematic review. Pediatr Emerg Care 2018;34(8):594–8.
121. Hendrickson JE, Shaz BH, Pereira G, et al. Coagulopathy is prevalent and associated with adverse outcomes in transfused pediatric trauma patients. J Pediatr 2012;160(2):204–9.e3.
122. Williams MD, Chalmers EA, Gibson BE, Haemostasis and Thrombosis Task Force, British Committee for Standards in Haematology. The investigation and management of neonatal haemostasis and thrombosis. Br J Haematol 2002; 119(2):295–309.
123. Schulte R, Jordan LC, Morad A, et al. Rise in late onset vitamin K deficiency bleeding in young infants because of omission or refusal of prophylaxis at birth. Pediatr Neurol 2014;50(6):564–8.
124. Shearer MJ. Vitamin K deficiency bleeding (VKDB) in early infancy. Blood Rev 2009;23(2):49–59.
125. Padmanabhan A, Connelly-Smith L, Aqui N, et al. Guidelines on the use of therapeutic Apheresis in clinical practice - evidence-based approach from the writing committee of the American Society for Apheresis: the eighth special issue. J Clin Apher 2019;34(3):171–354.
126. New HV, Stanworth SJ, Engelfriet CP, et al. Neonatal transfusions. Vox Sang 2009;96(1):62–85.
127. Eaton MP, Iannoli EM. Coagulation considerations for infants and children undergoing cardiopulmonary bypass. Paediatr Anaesth 2011;21(1):31–42.
128. Mou SS, Giroir BP, Molitor-Kirsch EA, et al. Fresh whole blood versus reconstituted blood for pump priming in heart surgery in infants. N Engl J Med 2004; 351(16):1635–44.

129. Gruenwald CE, McCrindle BW, Crawford-Lean L, et al. Reconstituted fresh whole blood improves clinical outcomes compared with stored component blood therapy for neonates undergoing cardiopulmonary bypass for cardiac surgery: a randomized controlled trial. J Thorac Cardiovasc Surg 2008;136(6): 1442–9.
130. Miao X, Liu J, Zhao M, et al. Evidence-based use of FFP: the influence of a priming strategy without FFP during CPB on postoperative coagulation and recovery in pediatric patients. Perfusion 2015;30(2):140–7.
131. Miao X, Liu J, Zhao M, et al. The influence of cardiopulmonary bypass priming without FFP on postoperative coagulation and recovery in pediatric patients with cyanotic congenital heart disease. Eur J Pediatr 2014;173(11):1437–43.
132. Christensen RD, Baer VL, Lambert DK, et al. Reference intervals for common coagulation tests of preterm infants (CME). Transfusion 2014;54(3):627–32 [quiz: 626].
133. Naderi M, Tabibian S, Alizadeh S, et al. Congenital factor V deficiency: comparison of the severity of clinical presentations among patients with rare bleeding disorders. Acta Haematol 2015;133(2):148–54.
134. Huang JN, Koerper MA. Factor V deficiency: a concise review. Haemophilia 2008;14(6):1164–9.

Massive Transfusion in Pediatric Patients

Lucas P. Neff, MD[a],*, Michael Aaron Beckwith, MD[b], Robert T. Russell, MD, MPH[c], Jeremy W. Cannon, MD, MA[d], Philip C. Spinella, MD[e]

KEYWORDS

- Pediatric massive transfusion • Hemorrhage • Blood failure • Whole blood
- Endotheliopathy

KEY POINTS

- A universal definition of massive transfusion in children remains elusive. The definitions are typically based on the volume of blood products transfused as a function of the estimated total blood volume of a child given over a given period of time.
- Pediatric transfusions carry a spectrum of risks similar to adult transfusions. These risks include metabolic derangements, coagulation dysregulation, immunologic reactions, volume disturbances, or any combination of effects.
- The optimal ratio of blood products transfused in pediatric patients has its basis in the adult trauma literature. Several studies have evaluated the benefit of a balanced resuscitation in children without a clear survival advantage, but more investigation is needed.
- The resurgence of whole blood for adult trauma resuscitation has renewed interests in its application in the pediatric realm. The primary concerns are its possible allogeneic reactions and its overall availability. More evidence showing its safety and effectiveness is emerging.
- Pharmacologic adjuncts to resuscitation (eg, tranexamic acid and recombinant factor VIIa) should be considered in severely bleeding children. Thromboelastography and rotational thromboelastometry are two tests that can be used at the point of care to guide treatment of coagulopathy.

[a] Department of General Surgery, Section of Pediatric Surgery, Wake Forest University School of Medicine, 5th Floor, Watlington Hall, Medical Center Boulevard, Winston-Salem, NC 27157, USA; [b] Division of Trauma and Acute Care Surgery, Department of Surgery, University of Alabama at Birmingham, 1922 7th Avenue South, KB 120, Birmingham, AL 35294, USA; [c] Pediatric General Surgery, Division of Pediatric Surgery, Department of Surgery, University of Alabama at Birmingham, 1600 7th Avenue South, Lowder, Suite 300, Birmingham, AL 35233, USA; [d] Division of Traumatology, Surgical Critical Care, and Emergency Surgery, Department of Surgery, Perelman School of Medicine at the University of Pennsylvania, Penn Presbyterian Medical Center, 51 North 39th Street, Suite 120 MOB, Philadelphia, PA 19104, USA; [e] Division of Critical Care Medicine, Department of Pediatrics, The Washington University of Saint Louis, 4905 Children's Place, St Louis, MO 63110, USA
* Corresponding author.
E-mail address: lpneff@wakehealth.edu
Twitter: @lpneff (L.P.N.)

Clin Lab Med 41 (2021) 35–49
https://doi.org/10.1016/j.cll.2020.10.003
0272-2712/21/© 2020 Elsevier Inc. All rights reserved.

INTRODUCTION

Life-threatening hemorrhage (LTH) in children is a rare but potentially catastrophic event. The timely delivery of blood products can mean the difference between life and death. Although the term massive transfusion has been used to describe the phenomenon of large-volume delivery of blood products to an exsanguinating child, an accurate definition that is clearly linked to outcomes remains elusive. Moreover, the term massive can be misleading in children for whom small absolute volumes of blood loss can invoke significant physiologic derangements. This article focuses on the pathophysiology of hemorrhagic shock from injury and the current practice of hemostatic resuscitation in children.

EPIDEMIOLOGY OF LIFE-THREATENING HEMORRHAGE IN CHILDREN

Injury is the leading cause of death in children and adolescents, with falls and motor vehicle accidents as the two leading mechanisms of injury.[1,2] Bleeding from these mechanisms can be severe enough to warrant massive transfusion protocol activations. Additional causes of LTH include surgical bleeding and gastrointestinal bleeding.[3–6] Despite these varied reasons for hemorrhage, traumatic injury accounts for most activations of pediatric massive transfusion protocols. This subset of patients with trauma is generally older, more hypothermic, and has a higher injury severity score compared with other pediatric patients with trauma who were transfused but did not meet the criteria for pediatric massive transfusion.[7]

However, pediatric massive transfusion protocol activation is an uncommon event. From 2010 to 2012, 13,523 (4%) of the 356,583 pediatric patients in the National Trauma Data Bank required any amount of blood product transfusion within 24 hours of injury. Of that group, only 173 children (0.04%) required a massive transfusion, defined as 40 mL/kg within the first 24 hours.[7] Although it is comforting that this is a low number of pediatric patients with trauma, it is likely an underestimate, and the paucity of data prevents a broader perspective on the specific issues highlighted by this article. In addition to children and adolescents, neonates represent a special subset of the pediatric patient population that may require massive transfusion by virtue of the small amount of absolute blood loss that they can tolerate before profound shock results.[6]

The epidemiology, therapies commonly used, and outcomes related to severe hemorrhage have not been systematically studied in children. As such, there is a major knowledge gap in this population. The Massive Transfusion in Children (MATIC) study sought to better understand indications, frequency, therapies, and outcomes for 481 children with LTH in a prospective observational study. Children were categorized as having traumatic injury, operative, or medical bleeding as the cause of the LTH. Children with traumatic LTH have a 28-day mortality ranging from 37% to 50%[7] (Phillip Spinella, unpublished data from the MATIC study, 2020), which is 200% higher than the 20% to 24% observed in adults with traumatic LTH. Morbidity is also very high in children with traumatic LTH. Post-LTH, 21% of these children develop acute respiratory distress syndrome, and 20% experience renal failure.[8]

Preliminary results from the MATIC study suggest the most common cause of LTH was trauma. The transfusion ratio (milliliters per kilogram transfused) of plasma relative to red cells of greater than 1:2 in children with LTH from both traumatic injury and operative bleeding was independently associated with improved 24-hour survival. In all causes of LTH, the use of crystalloid was approximately 22% of the total milliliters per kilogram of blood and fluids administered during resuscitation. The administration of intravenous hemostatic adjuncts was uncommon, with recombinant factor VIIa (rFVIIa) most commonly used in 12% of the cohort. The overall 24-hour mortality after the LTH event was 21.6% for all children (trauma, 25%; operative, 9.9%; medical, 35.1%)[8] (Phillip Spinella, unpublished data from the MATIC study, 2020).

Trauma-Induced Blood Failure

In both adults and children, approximately 25% to 35% of severely injured patients with trauma presenting with severe anatomic injuries develop shock and coagulopathy.[9,10] Hypoperfusion of the microvasculature and tissues causes shock or oxygen debt. When shock is combined with traumatic injury, the result is endothelial cell damage, which causes inflammation and hemostatic dysfunction. Both blood and the endothelium act as organs. Thus, when there is dysfunction that causes reduced delivery of oxygen with impaired endothelial, immune, and hemostatic function, it is instructive to consider this interconnected pathophysiology under the term trauma-induced blood failure.[11,12] The term blood failure serves as a reminder that blood is an organ, and, when it is dysfunctional, the entire system should be considered when therapies are indicated to achieve balance and improve function.[13] Trauma-induced blood failure is initiated by blood loss, which leads to decreased preload and reduced cardiac output that causes systemic oxygen delivery to decrease to levels insufficient for aerobic metabolism. The shock that occurs when oxygen delivery does not meet metabolic demands leads to altered blood redox potential, lactic acidosis, and an increase in adrenergic mediators, including epinephrine.[14] The cascade of effects on the endothelium, plasma proteins, blood cells, and immune system constitute the endotheliopathy, coagulopathy, and immune dysfunction that represents blood failure. This process subsequently can be exacerbated by plasma dilution, hypothermia, acidosis, and further consumption of coagulation factors and platelets.

To appropriately treat trauma-induced blood failure, interventions must simultaneously address the multiple components. Treatment of the oxygen debt, endothelial injury, and coagulopathy should occur concurrently. Packed red blood cells (PRBCs) are given to primarily address oxygen debt along with improving intravascular volume and subsequently cardiac output. Plasma transfusion also supports cardiac output through intravascular volume expansion, provides coagulation factors, and may provide some degree of endothelial protection and repair based on animal studies.[15,16] Early platelet transfusions can contribute to hemostasis in bleeding patients with trauma by increasing thrombin formation, promoting enhanced clot stiffness, and increasing resistance to clot lysis, and may also improve endothelial repair.[17-19] Cryoprecipitate provides a rich source of fibrinogen, factor VIII, and von Willebrand factor. The benefits from cryoprecipitate can be seen in improved viscoelastic clot strength with early and aggressive supplementation.[20] In addition, fresh whole blood and cold-stored whole blood have reemerged as therapies that potentially can simultaneously address multiple critical components of blood failure. Oxygen debt, endotheliopathy, and coagulopathy may all be addressed by whole-blood transfusion with approximately 300% less volume of anticoagulant and additive solutions relative to the use of component therapy in a 1:1:1-unit ratio. Preliminary data with both fresh whole blood and cold-stored low-titer O whole blood suggest that the use of whole blood may improve 24-hour, 28-day, and in-hospital survival compared with individual blood component therapy.[21-23]

DEFINITION OF MASSIVE TRANSFUSION IN CHILDREN

Over the last several years, multiple pediatric studies have attempted to define massive transfusion in the pediatric population as the initial step toward developing prediction tools and refining protocols using retrospective datasets. This difficulty in a universal definition is apparent in the adult transfusion literature as well, with multiple competing definitions of massive transfusion, all seeking to adequately describe this patient population.[24,25] This attempt to create a standardized definition as an indicator of increased risk of death from hemorrhage has been limited by the heterogeneity of patient populations studied and the difficulty in acquiring the granularity of detail required to adequately account for all potential confounders between transfusion requirements and mortality.[26–28]

As such, many pediatric massive transfusion definitions are based on the volume of blood products transfused as a function of the estimated total blood volume for the child over a 4-hour, 12-hour, or 24-hour period.[29–33] A recent study of children treated in a combat environment indicated that 40 mL/kg transfused within a 24-hour period yielded the highest sensitivity and specificity for identifying critically injured children at risk for death at any point after 24 hours.[30] Given a 24-hour time frame, the introduction of lead-time (ie, survival) bias may have confounded findings because some children did not survive long enough to meet a 40 mL/kg/24 h threshold. In addition, the predominance of blast and other penetrating mechanisms of injury in this study may not have external validity in children with blunt injury, which is much more common in civilian settings.[3,30] To limit survival bias and define massive transfusion in a more representative pediatric trauma population, a recent Trauma Quality Improvement Project (TQIP) study of civilian patients with trauma with and without traumatic brain injury found that this same mortality threshold existed above the 37 mL/kg/4 h time point[33] (**Table 1**).

INDICATIONS FOR MASSIVE TRANSFUSION PROTOCOL ACTIVATION

Massive transfusion protocol activation often occurs emergently and without notice. Given that blood product delivery and transfusion is a highly regulated and laborious process, it requires some lead time. Thus, the ability to rapidly predict massive transfusion protocol activation ahead of its need is an area of great interest in the trauma community. Multiple rapid scoring systems have been devised in the adult transfusion literature to predict the need for massive transfusion protocol activation.[28,34,35] These rapid prognostic systems rely on admission physiologic parameters, laboratory values, associated injuries, and cause of hemorrhage. Moreover, these scoring systems were developed in the context of hemorrhage from traumatic injury. In all cases, these prediction scoring systems are validated by multiple follow-up studies. For children, no such tool exists that takes into account the differences in physiology and common injury patterns that predominate in pediatric trauma. However, the ideal pediatric massive transfusion prognostic tool capturing prehospital or admission hemodynamic variables would be simple and should integrate automatically within the workflow of the resuscitation team. At present, validated scoring systems for children have only mortality prediction capabilities rather than a prediction of the need for massive transfusion.[36]

For most pediatric hospitals, the decision to activate the massive transfusion protocol is at the discretion of the clinician. Because massive transfusions are an uncommon event in children, using clinical judgment in an ad hoc fashion can lead to inconsistent use and ineffective transfusion or blood product mismanagement. In an effort to improve the quality of massive transfusion protocol implementation, some pediatric centers have simply designated every high-acuity trauma activation as the single criterion for the release of the first packet (red cells, plasma, platelets) of blood products.[37] Other centers have taken a more selective approach by requiring the patient to fail the initial crystalloid challenge as a partial or nonresponder before

Table 1
Definitions of massive transfusion in pediatric literature

Author	Population	Definition of Massive Transfusion	Strengths	Limitations
Nosanov et al,[28] 2013	Pediatric patients with trauma who received blood within 24 h	>50% of patient's blood volume transfused within 24 h	Large cohort identified over several years at a large, US pediatric trauma center	Includes children with head injuries, which can obscure any mortality benefit from transfusion
Neff et al,[29] 2015	Department of Defense Joint Theater Trauma Registry	Transfusion ≥40 mL/kg of all blood products in 24 h	Burns, drowning, isolated head injuries, and patients without an injury severity score were excluded	Children with combat injuries with blast and penetrating trauma predominating; 24-h totals of blood products
Horst et al,[30] 2016	Survey of 46 pediatric massive transfusion protocols	Institution based, examples are >40 mL/kg in 2 h, >50% of blood volume in 2 h, and continued need for transfusion	Broad response, multiple variables, including ratios, hemostatic agents, massive transfusion protocol activation, and compliance	Limited response from surveyed institutions by a variety of individuals with varying pediatric massive transfusion protocol experience
Cannon et al,[31] 2017	Department of Defense Joint Theater Trauma Registry	Transfusion ≥40 mL/kg in 24 h	Burns, drowning, and isolated head injuries and patients aged ≥18 y were excluded	Children with combat injuries were the only ones reviewed. The mechanism of injury is not as applicable in developed countries
Cunningham et al,[32] 2019	Pediatric TQIP data	Transfusion ≥40 mL/kg in 24 h	Large cohort, multi-institution dataset; burns, dead on arrival and nonsurvivable injuries excluded	Retrospective, limited by data in the TQIP database

activating the massive transfusion protocol.[38] Given the paucity of data regarding which children need massive transfusion, simple and straightforward criteria are the most likely to ensure timely access to blood products. Further investigation to establish novel pediatric-specific prediction algorithms or validate the existing adult criteria for children is needed.

COMPLICATIONS OF MASSIVE TRANSFUSION

As in the adult population, massive transfusion in a pediatric patient carries significant risk of complications. These risks include electrolyte abnormalities, transfusion reactions (immunogenic and nonimmunogenic), hemodilution, volume overload, or a combination of effects. These complications can range from being asymptomatic to fatal. As a result, they must be carefully monitored and rapidly addressed if they occur in a child with life-threatening bleeding.

The most common complications of a massive transfusion event, regardless of age, are metabolic disturbances. Among these, posttransfusion hypocalcemia predominates because of the chelation of calcium by the citrate anticoagulant in blood components. Although important for all children, this issue is extremely pertinent to the neonatal population. These patients have a decreased ability to metabolize citrate, and hypocalcemia reduces cardiac contractility; which is the primary compensatory mechanism to increase cardiac output in neonates. Hypocalcemia prevention for this group includes prophylactic intravenous calcium.[38]

The second most common electrolyte disturbance is hyperkalemia, which arises from the leakage of intracellular potassium into the additive solution and plasma during component storage. Because most blood banks practice a first in, first out policy for blood products, the consequence is that even children with LTH receive the oldest red blood cell (RBC) units in the inventory, increasing the risk of hyperkalemia.[39] Posttransfusion hyperkalemia has been implicated in fatal cardiac arrhythmias in pediatric massive transfusion events. Measures to reduce transfusion-related hyperkalemia include the use of large-bore intravascular catheters to prevent hemolysis with the transfusion of RBCs, the use of blood warmers specifically validated for large-volume rapid blood transfusion, monitoring of potassium levels, and the use of the freshest RBCs in the blood bank where available.[40]

Other complications of massive transfusion include hemodilution and citrate toxicity secondary to anticoagulant chelation of the ionized fraction of plasma calcium. When individual blood components are transfused compared with a whole-blood unit, there is a significant amount of hemodilution and increased exposure to citrate anticoagulation. For example, 6 units of whole blood contains approximately 360 to 420 mL of anticoagulant-preservative or additive solution, whereas 6 units of PRBCs contain greater than 700 mL of anticoagulant-preservative or additive solution, 6 units of fresh frozen plasma (FFP) contain 300 mL, and 1 unit of apheresis platelets contains 35 mL (**Table 2**).[41] Thus, transfusing blood components in a 1:1:1 unit ratio exposes the patient to approximately 3 times the amount of additive solution and anticoagulant compared with the equivalent volume of whole blood.[41]

RATIOS OF BLOOD PRODUCTS

The highest-quality evidence for optimal blood product ratios arises from the adult trauma literature and several prospective observational trials arising from the US military combat medicine experience in Iraq and Afghanistan.[42–44] These findings informed much of the pediatric care in those combat zones and have influenced the civilian population by extension.

Table 2
Comparing whole blood with component therapy

	Whole Blood	Component Therapy (1 PRBC, 1 PLT, 1 FFP, 1 Cryo)
Volume (mL)	500	680
Hematocrit (%)	38–50	29
Platelets (per μL)	150,000–440,000	80,000
Coagulation factors (%)	100	65

Abbreviations: Cryo, cryoprecipitate; PLT, platelets.

In 2007, Borgman and colleagues[44] published a retrospective study of combat massive transfusion data in adults that compared FFP/PRBC median ratios of 1:8, 1:2.5, and 1:1.4 and found that the high ratio relative to FFP transfused, 1:1.4, was independently associated with improved survival.[45] This finding was subsequently confirmed by reports in the civilian population.[46] These initial studies paved the way for prospective trials to determine optimal ratios of blood components for patients with life-threatening bleeding.

Two large-scale controlled prospective clinical trials in adult patients with trauma were the Prospective Observational Multicenter Major Trauma Transfusion (PROMMTT) and the Pragmatic Randomized Optimal Platelet and FFP Ratios (PROPPR) trials. PROMMTT included 10 level I trauma centers in the United States and prospectively reviewed time to transfusion and ratios given during massive transfusion. The study concluded that a higher ratio of FFP and platelet administration to red cells decreased mortality in patients who received at least 3 units of blood products in the first 24 hours. In the first 6 hours, patients with ratios less than 1:2 FFP/PRBCs had increased mortality. However, after the first 24 hours, ratios did not correlate with mortality risk.[47] PROPPR was a randomized controlled trial that evaluated an FFP/platelet/PRBC ratio of 1:1:1 compared with 1:1:2 in patients needing massive transfusion at 12 level I trauma centers in North America over a 16-month period. The PROPPR trial found no difference in overall mortality but decreased death by exsanguination at 24 hours and increased achievement of hemostasis in the 1:1:1 group. Complication rates were high in both groups (87.9% in the 1:1:1 vs 90.6% in the 1:1:2 group) and were widely varied to include systemic inflammatory response syndrome, deep vein thrombosis, and infection, to name a few.[48]

These landmark trials provided the clinical rationale to subsequently investigate the benefits of a balanced transfusion in pediatric patients with trauma. Cannon and colleagues[31] studied pediatric patients with trauma from the Department of Defense (DOD) Trauma Registry from the years 2001 to 2013. This study defined massive transfusion as greater than or equal to 40 mL/kg total blood products in 24 hours and concluded that a high FFP/PRBC ratio ($\geq$1:2) did not confer survival.[32] In 2019, Cunningham and colleagues[32] published a retrospective review of the Pediatric TQIP database studying low (<1:2), medium ($\geq$1:2, <1:1), and high ($\geq$1:1) FFP and platelet to PRBC ratios. This TQIP review found a survival benefit in the high-ratio group with regard to FFP, low versus medium versus high, at 4 hours (14% vs 14% vs 2%, $P<.01$) and at 24 hours (23% vs 24% vs 12%, $P = .02$). They found no difference with platelet groups.[33] Noland and colleagues[48] in 2019 also reported a survival benefit with a 1:1 PRBC/FFP ratio in pediatric patients receiving massive transfusion.[49] As of 2020, the largest observational study of blood product ratios included nearly 600 children from the TQIP database and reported a 51% (adjusted relative risk, 0.49; 95% confidence interval [CI], 0.27–0.87) decrease in mortality following resuscitation using high (>1:1

FFP/PRBC) ratios compared with low (<1:2 FFP/PRBC) ratios. However, this mortality reduction was again not seen with higher platelet/PRBC ratios.[50] In the absence of high-quality prospective observational trials with pediatric massive transfusion, these retrospective analyses are the current best evidence to support the use of at least 1:1 FFP/RBC ratios in pediatric massive transfusion protocols. A review of the pediatric resuscitation practices using data from US military care facilities in combat operations revealed a shift toward increased use of balanced hemostatic resuscitation (increased plasma and platelets relative to red cells) and that mortality decreased over time in pediatric patients who received massive transfusion with these ratios.[51] These data from military operations provide additional support for the implementation of balanced resuscitation in children who required massive transfusion from LTH.

BARRIERS TO MASSIVE TRANSFUSION PROTOCOL ADHERENCE AND IMPLEMENTATION

The infrequent nature of pediatric massive transfusion poses a challenge in creating, implementing, standardizing, and evaluating pediatric massive transfusion protocols. However, this standardizing for quality assurance (QA) requires precise definitions of terms. Pediatric massive transfusion protocol activation must be defined as a discrete binary event; it is either activated or not. Because this is not always the situation with pediatric trauma resuscitation, there are many challenges that face QA teams in evaluation of, adherence to, and implementation of pediatric massive transfusion protocols.

These processes can be further subdivided into systems issues and factors unique to each particular trauma resuscitation. Common systems issues include lack of standardized formatting for recording sheets for massive transfusion or simply a failure to document the massive transfusion protocol activation at all. There is also a lack of knowledge among practitioners about transfusion-related complications, transfusion event tracking, blood warmers, high-volume rapid transfusion devices, intravenous and topical hemostatic agents, harmful effects of crystalloids, and transient periods of hypertension that may impair clot formation in arterial lesions. The Broxton MTP Massive Transfusion Protocol Evaluation Tool was created to standardize and collect information regarding massive transfusion protocol activations to improve the QA process.[52] Identified barriers were primarily caused by deficiencies in the electronic medical record and a need to streamline data entry during massive transfusion protocol activation. There was also no electronic medical record workspace for documentation of massive transfusions, making attempts at retrospective QA review challenging. Horst and colleagues[30] in 2016 analyzed 46 pediatric massive transfusion protocols identifying common challenges.[31] Fifty-three percent of centers with a pediatric massive transfusion protocol had a 1:1 FFP/PRBC ratio established for the first round of resuscitation. The obstacles to a balanced resuscitation in the portion of hospitals not using a 1:1 ratio included limited availability of FFP. Although 89% of responding pediatric trauma centers had emergency release type-O PRBCs immediately available, less than half (48%) of centers had thawed FFP or liquid plasma. The logistical constraints of providing recently thawed FFP at pediatric centers loom large, which is why many trauma centers maintain an inventory of liquid plasma and whole blood. Nationwide, pediatric massive transfusion knowledge is still growing. Robust data collection and analysis will be necessary before more evidence-based best-practice recommendations can be possible. At present, the small numbers of study subjects can lead to erroneous conclusions about the ultimate morbidity and mortality benefit of any 1 practice. For example, a literature review of outcomes before and after implementation of a pediatric massive transfusion protocol found no difference in mortality despite the postprotocol patients receiving a higher ratio of platelets to RBCs. However, it is difficult to make any meaningful conclusion on data that encapsulate only 43 patients over 9 years.[53]

WHOLE BLOOD

The increasing adoption of whole-blood transfusion during the last 2 decades by the United States military during combat operations has resulted in a robust experience of children treated in military facilities using this product.[30,51] As such, there is renewed interest in the use of whole blood in the pediatric trauma population, whereas whole blood was previously largely relegated to adults.

In adults, the use of low-titer group-O whole blood (LTOWB) for traumatic LTH has reemerged in clinical practice. Approximately 70 medical centers in the United States use LTOWB for LTH (A.B. Nathens MD MPH PhD, personal communication, 2020). Data from multiple adult retrospective and prospective observational studies of traumatic LTH indicate the use of LTOWB compared with component therapy (CT) (red cells, plasma, and platelets) is associated with improved oxygen delivery and mortality at both 24 hours and 28 days.[22] Benefits of LTOWB compared with individual components for LTH include improved oxygen delivery and hemostatic function, lower risk of fatal hemolytic reactions and bacterial contamination, and more rapid administration.[54,55] As a result, there is the potential for LTOWB compared with individual blood components to more effectively reverse oxygen deficits, hemostatic dysfunction, and endothelial dysfunction, and improve outcomes.[55]

The use of LTOWB for children is less common than in adults, but it is currently in use for traumatic bleeding in at least 12 institutions (Phillip Spinella, unpublished data from the MATIC study, 2020) Data from 2 pediatric studies indicate that the use of LTOWB compared with CT both reduces the median time from admission of transfusing red cells, plasma, and platelets by more than 4 hours and improves clearance of base deficit, which is a surrogate for oxygen delivery.[56,57] Initial reports of pediatric whole blood transfusion during trauma bay resuscitation indicate that up to 20 mL/kg of warm whole blood administered as the initial transfusion is safe and effective.[57] This experience with 18 patients greater than 15 kg from the Children's Hospital of Pittsburgh allowed efficient delivery of whole blood within 15 minutes of arrival without any transfusion-related complications. In addition, concerns of platelet dysfunction arising from cold storage of the whole blood have not been backed up in early reports.[58]

A significant concern with increasing whole blood use is recipient hemolysis caused by anti-A or anti-B antibodies contained in the plasma component of the whole blood unit when transfused to a non–type-O recipient. As of 2020, it is still unclear how clinically significant this phenomenon is and what the overall risk to a given patient might be. To mitigate this risk, many adult trauma centers transfuse LTOWB. Use of LTOWB resulted in no increased hemolysis and is showing promise in children as well.[58] However, there are currently no national standards as to what constitutes an acceptable low titer in the pediatric population.

In clinical practice, LTOWB seems to be safe, effective, and has logistic benefits compared with the use of individual blood components during an emergency massive transfusion event, possibly because rapidly and massively bleeding patients bleed out their incompatible non-O red cells in addition to any other alloantibodies in their plasma, which are replaced with the donor LTOWB, effectively creating a whole-blood exchange. It is reasonable to consider the use of LTOWB in nonneonatal pediatric massive transfusion protocols while clinical trials are underway to more thoroughly examine these outcomes.[59]

ADJUNCTS

As with the blood product ratio concept for pediatric resuscitation, there is a paucity of quality data to guide the use of intravenous hemostatic adjuncts such as tranexamic acid and recombinant factor VIIa in children. Future research is needed to include outcomes when both a balanced transfusion strategy and adjuncts are used together. This combination may address the hyperfibrinolysis and coagulopathy following massive hemorrhage.

Tranexamic acid (TXA) is a thoroughly studied and used lysine analogue that prevents fibrinolysis by inhibiting plasminogen activation. This plasminogen inhibition prevents development of plasmin and subsequent breakdown of fibrin, thus preventing clot disruption. Multiple studies in both civilian and military trauma populations have provided only modest results.[60,61] However, the successful use of TXA in Operation Enduring Freedom prompted health care providers to extend this practice beyond children injured by war. The PED-TRAX (Pediatric Trauma and Tranexamic Acid) study evaluated pediatric patients with trauma with predominantly blast or penetrating injury mechanisms who received TXA as part of their massive hemorrhage resuscitations.[62] Approximately 10% of the pediatric patients with trauma in this study were administered TXA, which was found to be independently associated with a decrease in mortality (odds ratio, 0.27; 95% CI, 0.85–0.89), and there were no adverse effects identified with its use in this study. However, the results in a civilian trauma population may not show the same benefit and might carry an increased risk for nonhemorrhage neurologic complications.[63,64] A meta-analysis of 2 large randomized controlled trials in adults with acute bleeding reported that TXA administration had no statistically significant worse outcomes compared with placebo or increased incidence of adverse events.[65] Several additional translational studies further evaluated intraosseous administration of TXA in a porcine model and discovered that intraosseous and intravenous TXA had similar bioavailability and efficacy.[66,67] Based on these studies, use of TXA should be considered in pediatric massive hemorrhage protocols.

In addition to TXA, several studies have suggested recombinant factor VIIa for the reversal of profound coagulopathy in patients needing massive transfusion with less volume than FFP.[68] However, even with the suggestion that rFVIIa may decrease overall blood component usage during resuscitation without increased venous thromboembolism formation, the data for empiric administration to bleeding patients are limited and do not include the pediatric population. As such, rFVIIa incorporation into pediatric massive transfusion protocols is not yet recommended.

Although TXA and rFVIIa have the potential to be useful adjuncts, point-of-care coagulation testing to guide administration of blood products has clear evidence-based practice potential. Thromboelastography (TEG) and rotational thromboelastometry (ROTEM) are two blood testing platforms that are now widely used in the adult trauma population.[69] Often patients who require massive transfusion are hemorrhaging at a rate that exceeds the utility of typical laboratory studies to guide product administration because coagulation and hematology measurements have a lag time from bleed to change in laboratory value. TEG and ROTEM provide real-time feedback to guide product administration and can identify the development of hyperfibrinolysis, prompting antifibrinolytic countermeasures such as TXA. Although TEG and ROTEM parameters are available for pediatric patients, their use is not mainstream in pediatric massive transfusion despite demonstrated benefit in adult patients with trauma.[70,71]

Careful consideration should be given to the implementation of TEG and ROTEM in pediatric massive transfusion protocols, and further research is needed to determine its true efficacy for children.

FUTURE DIRECTIONS

There are ample opportunities for research of optimal methods to resuscitate children with life-threatening bleeding and to determine how to best use massive transfusion protocols. One example is the call for a national focus to improve the implementation and standardization of massive transfusion protocols in children.[72] As the field moves forward, it will be important to consider the common biases and pitfalls of transfusion outcomes research in order to mitigate these and produce the most critical conclusions. Although guidelines and recommendations are coming into focus for adults, in pediatrics there is still a great deal yet to be discovered.

DISCLOSURE

P.C. Spinella: consultant for Secure Transfusion Services, Cerus, and Octapharma. J.W. Cannon: DOD funding on resuscitation/decision support, UpToDate royalties on REBOA (resuscitative endovascular balloon occlusion of the aorta). The other authors have nothing to disclose.

REFERENCES

1. Dzik WH, Blajchman MA, Fergusson D, et al. Clinical review: Canadian National Advisory Committee on blood and blood products–massive transfusion consensus conference 2011: report of the panel. Crit Care 2011;15(6):242.
2. Stewart RM, Nathens AB, Chang MC. 2016:128 NTDB Reports and Publications. American College of Surgeons. Available at: https://www.facs.org/quality-programs/trauma/tqp/center-programs/ntdb/docpub. Accessed May 2, 2020.
3. Edwards MJ, Lustik M, Eichelberger MR, et al. Blast injury in children: an analysis from Afghanistan and Iraq, 2002-2010. J Trauma Acute Care Surg 2012;73(5): 1278–83.
4. Tasker RC, Turgeon AF, Spinella PC, Pediatric critical care Transfusion and Anemia Expertise Initiative (TAXI), Pediatric Critical Care Blood Research Network (BloodNet), and the Pediatric Acute Lung Injury and Sepsis Investigators (PALISI) Network. Recommendations on RBC transfusion in critically III children with acute brain injury from the pediatric critical care transfusion and anemia expertise initiative. Pediatr Crit Care Med 2018;19(9S Suppl 1):S133–6.
5. Paterson NA. Validation of a theoretically derived model for the management of massive blood loss in pediatric patients - a case report. Paediatr Anaesth 2009;19(5):535–40.
6. Diab YA, Wong ECC, Luban NLC. Massive transfusion in children and neonates. Br J Haematol 2013;161(1):15–26.
7. Shroyer MC, Griffin RL, Mortellaro VE, et al. Massive transfusion in pediatric trauma: analysis of the National Trauma Databank. J Surg Res 2017;208:166–72.
8. Niles SE, McLaughlin DF, Perkins JG, et al. Increased mortality associated with the early coagulopathy of trauma in combat casualties. J Trauma 2008;64(6): 1459–63 [discussion: 1463–5].
9. Patregnani JT, Borgman MA, Maegele M, et al. Coagulopathy and shock on admission is associated with mortality for children with traumatic injuries at combat support hospitals. Pediatr Crit Care Med 2012;13(3):273–7.

10. Cannon JW. Hemorrhagic shock. N Engl J Med 2018;378(4):370–9.
11. White NJ, Ward KR, Pati S, et al. Hemorrhagic blood failure: oxygen debt, coagulopathy, and endothelial damage. J Trauma Acute Care Surg 2017;82(6S Suppl 1):S41–9.
12. Spinella PC, Trauma Hemostasis and Oxygenation Research Network. Damage control resuscitation: identification and treatment of life-threatening hemorrhage; 2020. Available at: https://www.springer.com/gp/book/9783030208196.
13. Johansson PI, Ostrowski SR. Acute coagulopathy of trauma: balancing progressive catecholamine induced endothelial activation and damage by fluid phase anticoagulation. Med Hypotheses 2010;75(6):564–7.
14. Kozar RA, Peng Z, Zhang R, et al. Plasma restoration of endothelial glycocalyx in a rodent model of hemorrhagic shock. Anesth Analg 2011;112(6):1289–95.
15. Lawless RA, Holcomb JB. Plasma Transfusion. In: Gonzalez E, Moore H, Moore E, editors. Trauma Induced Coagulopathy. Springer, Cham; 2016. https://doi.org/10.1007/978-3-319-28308-1_20.
16. Cardenas JC, Zhang X, Fox EE, et al. Platelet transfusions improve hemostasis and survival in a substudy of the prospective, randomized PROPPR trial. Blood Adv 2018;2(14):1696–704.
17. Moore HB, Moore EE, Chapman MP, et al. Viscoelastic measurements of platelet function, not fibrinogen function, predicts sensitivity to tissue-type plasminogen activator in trauma patients. J Thromb Haemost 2015;13(10):1878–87.
18. Baimukanova G, Miyazawa B, Potter DR, et al. Platelets regulate vascular endothelial stability: assessing the storage lesion and donor variability of apheresis platelets. Transfusion (Paris) 2016;56(Suppl 1):S65–75.
19. Fries D, Martini WZ. Role of fibrinogen in trauma-induced coagulopathy. Br J Anaesth 2010;105(2):116–21.
20. Spinella PC, Perkins JG, Grathwohl KW, et al. Warm fresh whole blood is independently associated with improved survival for patients with combat-related traumatic injuries. J Trauma 2009;66(4 Suppl):S69–76.
21. Shea SM, Staudt AM, Thomas KA, et al. The use of low-titer group O whole blood is independently associated with improved survival compared to component therapy in adults with severe traumatic hemorrhage. Transfusion (Paris) 2020; 60(Suppl 3):S2–9.
22. Williams J, Merutka N, Meyer D, et al. Safety profile and impact of low-titer group O whole blood for emergency use in trauma. J Trauma Acute Care Surg 2020; 88(1):87–93.
23. Schuster KM, Davis KA, Lui FY, et al. The status of massive transfusion protocols in United States trauma centers: massive transfusion or massive confusion? Transfusion (Paris) 2010;50(7):1545–51.
24. Savage SA, Zarzaur BL, Croce MA, et al. Redefining massive transfusion when every second counts. J Trauma Acute Care Surg 2013;74(2):396–400 [discussion: 400–2].
25. Stanworth SJ, Morris TP, Gaarder C, et al. Reappraising the concept of massive transfusion in trauma. Crit Care 2010;14(6):R239.
26. Sihler KC, Napolitano LM. Massive transfusion: new insights. Chest 2009;136(6): 1654–67.
27. Rahbar E, Fox EE, del Junco DJ, et al. Early resuscitation intensity as a surrogate for bleeding severity and early mortality in the PROMMTT study. J Trauma Acute Care Surg 2013;75(1 Suppl 1):S16–23.
28. Nosanov L, Inaba K, Okoye O, et al. The impact of blood product ratios in massively transfused pediatric trauma patients. Am J Surg 2013;206(5):655–60.

29. Neff LP, Cannon JW, Morrison JJ, et al. Clearly defining pediatric massive transfusion: cutting through the fog and friction with combat data. J Trauma Acute Care Surg 2015;78(1):22–8 [discussion: 28–9].
30. Horst J, Leonard JC, Vogel A, et al. A survey of US and Canadian hospitals' paediatric massive transfusion protocol policies. Transfus Med 2016;26(1):49–56.
31. Cannon JW, Johnson MA, Caskey RC, et al. High ratio plasma resuscitation does not improve survival in pediatric trauma patients. J Trauma Acute Care Surg 2017;83(2):211–7.
32. Cunningham ME, Rosenfeld EH, Zhu H, et al. A high ratio of plasma: RBC improves survival in massively transfused injured children. J Surg Res 2019;233: 213–20.
33. Nunez TC, Voskresensky IV, Dossett LA, et al. Early prediction of massive transfusion in trauma: simple as ABC (assessment of blood consumption)? J Trauma 2009;66(2):346–52.
34. Shih AW, Al Khan S, Wang AY-H, et al. Systematic reviews of scores and predictors to trigger activation of massive transfusion protocols. J Trauma Acute Care Surg 2019;87(3):717–29.
35. Borgman MA, Maegele M, Wade CE, et al. Pediatric trauma BIG score: predicting mortality in children after military and civilian trauma. Pediatrics 2011;127(4): e892–7.
36. Hendrickson JE, Shaz BH, Pereira G, et al. Implementation of a pediatric trauma massive transfusion protocol: one institution's experience. Transfusion (Paris) 2012;52(6):1228–36.
37. Dehmer JJ, Adamson WT. Massive transfusion and blood product use in the pediatric trauma patient. Semin Pediatr Surg 2010;19(4):286–91.
38. Spinella PC, Dressler A, Tucci M, et al. Survey of transfusion policies at US and Canadian children's hospitals in 2008 and 2009. Transfusion (Paris) 2010; 50(11):2328–35.
39. Lee AC, Reduque LL, Luban NLC, et al. Transfusion-associated hyperkalemic cardiac arrest in pediatric patients receiving massive transfusion. Transfusion (Paris) 2014;54(1):244–54.
40. Murdock AD, Berséus O, Hervig T, et al. Whole blood: the future of traumatic hemorrhagic shock resuscitation. Shock 2014;41:62–9.
41. Borgman MA, Spinella PC, Holcomb JB, et al. The effect of FFP:RBC ratio on morbidity and mortality in trauma patients based on transfusion prediction score. Vox Sang 2011;101(1):44–54.
42. Spinella PC, Wade CE, Blackbourne LH, et al, Trauma Outcomes Group. The association of blood component use ratios with the survival of massively transfused trauma patients with and without severe brain injury. J Trauma 2011;71(2 Suppl 3):S343–52.
43. Cap AP, Spinella PC, Borgman MA, et al. Timing and location of blood product transfusion and outcomes in massively transfused combat casualties. J Trauma Acute Care Surg 2012;73(2 Suppl 1):S89–94.
44. Borgman MA, Spinella PC, Perkins JG, et al. The ratio of blood products transfused affects mortality in patients receiving massive transfusions at a combat support hospital. J Trauma 2007;63(4):805–13.
45. Spinella PC, Holcomb JB. Resuscitation and transfusion principles for traumatic hemorrhagic shock. Blood Rev 2009;23(6):231–40.
46. Holcomb JB, del Junco DJ, Fox EE, et al. The prospective, observational, multicenter, major trauma transfusion (PROMMTT) study: comparative effectiveness of a time-varying treatment with competing risks. JAMA Surg 2013;148(2):127–36.

47. Holcomb JB, Tilley BC, Baraniuk S, et al. Transfusion of plasma, platelets, and red blood cells in a 1:1:1 vs a 1:1:2 ratio and mortality in patients with severe trauma: the PROPPR randomized clinical trial. JAMA 2015;313(5):471–82.

48. Noland DK, Apelt N, Greenwell C, et al. Massive transfusion in pediatric trauma: an ATOMAC perspective. J Pediatr Surg 2019;54(2):345–9.

49. Butler EK, Mills BM, Arbabi S, et al. Association of blood component ratios with 24-hour mortality in injured children receiving massive transfusion. Crit Care Med 2019;47(7):975–83.

50. Cannon JW, Neff LP, Pidcoke HF, et al. The evolution of pediatric transfusion practice during combat operations 2001-2013. J Trauma Acute Care Surg 2018;84(6S Suppl 1):S69–76.

51. Broxton S, Medeiros R, Schumacher A. Evaluation tool for assessing a newly implemented massive transfusion protocol. J Trauma Nurs 2017;24(3):164–9.

52. Hwu RS, Spinella PC, Keller MS, et al. The effect of massive transfusion protocol implementation on pediatric trauma care. Transfusion (Paris) 2016;56(11):2712–9.

53. Mh Y, AP C, Pc S. Raising the standards on whole blood. J Trauma Acute Care Surg 2018;84(6S Suppl 1):S14–7.

54. Spinella PC, Gurney J, Yazer MH. Low titer group O whole blood for prehospital hemorrhagic shock: it is an offer we cannot refuse. Transfusion (Paris) 2019;59(7):2177–9.

55. Leeper CM, Neal MD, Billiar TR, et al. Overresuscitation with plasma is associated with sustained fibrinolysis shutdown and death in pediatric traumatic brain injury. J Trauma Acute Care Surg 2018;85(1):12–7.

56. Leeper CM, Yazer MH, Cladis FP, et al. Use of uncrossmatched cold-stored whole blood in injured children with hemorrhagic shock. JAMA Pediatr 2018;172(5):491–2.

57. Leeper CM, Yazer MH, Cladis FP, et al. Cold-stored whole blood platelet function is preserved in injured children with hemorrhagic shock. J Trauma Acute Care Surg 2019;87(1):49–53.

58. Leeper C, Yazer M, Triulzi D, et al. Whole blood is superior to component transfusion for injured children: a propensity matched analysis. Ann Surg 2020;272(4):590–4.

59. CRASH-2 Trial Collaborators, Shakur H, Roberts I, Bautista R, et al. Effects of tranexamic acid on death, vascular occlusive events, and blood transfusion in trauma patients with significant haemorrhage (CRASH-2): a randomised, placebo-controlled trial. Lancet 2010;376(9734):23–32.

60. Ramirez RJ, Spinella PC, Bochicchio GV. Tranexamic acid update in trauma. Crit Care Clin 2017;33(1):85–99.

61. Eckert MJ, Wertin TM, Tyner SD, et al. Tranexamic acid administration to pediatric trauma patients in a combat setting: the pediatric trauma and tranexamic acid study (PED-TRAX). J Trauma Acute Care Surg 2014;77(6):852–8 [discussion: 858].

62. Thomson JM, Huynh HH, Drone HM, et al. Experience in an urban level 1 trauma center with tranexamic acid in pediatric trauma: a retrospective chart review. J Intensive Care Med 2020. https://doi.org/10.1177/0885066619890834.

63. Maeda T, Michihata N, Sasabuchi Y, et al. Safety of tranexamic acid during pediatric trauma: a nationwide database study*. Pediatr Crit Care Med 2018;19(12):e637.

64. Ageron F-X, Gayet-Ageron A, Ker K, et al. Effect of tranexamic acid by baseline risk of death in acute bleeding patients: a meta-analysis of individual patient-level data from 28 333 patients. Br J Anaesth 2020;124(6):676–83.
65. Lallemand MS, Moe DM, McClellan JM, et al. No intravenous access, no problem: intraosseous administration of tranexamic acid is as effective as intravenous in a porcine hemorrhage model. J Trauma Acute Care Surg 2018;84(2):379–85.
66. Boysen SR, Pang JM, Mikler JR, et al. Comparison of tranexamic acid plasma concentrations when administered via intraosseous and intravenous routes. Am J Emerg Med 2017;35(2):227–33.
67. Boffard KD, Riou B, Warren B, et al. Recombinant factor VIIa as adjunctive therapy for bleeding control in severely injured trauma patients: two parallel randomized, placebo-controlled, double-blind clinical trials. J Trauma 2005;59(1):8–15 [discussion: 15–8].
68. Wikkelsø A, Wetterslev J, Møller AM, et al. Thromboelastography (TEG) or rotational thromboelastometry (ROTEM) to monitor haemostatic treatment in bleeding patients: a systematic review with meta-analysis and trial sequential analysis. Anaesthesia 2017;72(4):519–31.
69. Dias JD, Sauaia A, Achneck HE, et al. Thromboelastography-guided therapy improves patient blood management and certain clinical outcomes in elective cardiac and liver surgery and emergency resuscitation: a systematic review and analysis. J Thromb Haemost 2019;17(6):984–94.
70. Gonzalez E, Moore EE, Moore HB, et al. Goal-directed hemostatic resuscitation of trauma-induced coagulopathy: a pragmatic randomized clinical trial comparing a viscoelastic assay to conventional coagulation assays. Ann Surg 2016;263(6):1051–9.
71. Kamyszek RW, Leraas HJ, Reed C, et al. Massive transfusion in the pediatric population: a systematic review and summary of best-evidence practice strategies. J Trauma Acute Care Surg 2019;86(4):744–54.
72. del Junco DJ, Fox EE, Camp EA, et al, PROMMTT Study Group. Seven deadly sins in trauma outcomes research: an epidemiologic post mortem for major causes of bias. J Trauma Acute Care Surg 2013;75(1 Suppl 1):S97–103.

Pediatric Hemovigilance and Adverse Transfusion Reactions

Nataliya Sostin, MD, MCR[a,b], Jeanne E. Hendrickson, MD[a,b],*

KEYWORDS

- Transfusion reactions • Adverse reactions • Transfusion risks • Hemovigilance
- Serious hazards of transfusion • Neonate • Pediatrics

KEY POINTS

- Pediatric patients have a disproportionately high risk of transfusion reactions compared with adults.
- Allergic transfusion reactions are the most common reactions in children, with platelets being the component most likely to result in such reactions.
- Febrile nonhemolytic transfusion reactions are the second most common reactions in children, with more cases associated with red blood cells than any other blood products.
- Besides classic transfusion reactions, other posttransfusion sequelae should be considered in future studies in neonates and children.
- Collecting accurate statistics on pediatric transfusion reactions relies on hemovigilance systems, with some countries better equipped to gather these data than others.

INTRODUCTION

Pediatricians are taught very early in their training that neonates and children are not simply small adults. A large percentage of extremely low birth weight and very low birth weight neonates are transfused, with neonates accounting for between one-third and one-half of all pediatric transfusions.[1,2] The complexity of clinical presentation in combination with human errors, such as overtransfusion and a lack of knowledge about certain component modifications (eg, irradiation), affect transfusion outcomes in children.[3] Data from hemovigilance systems as well as single-center studies suggest that a disproportionate number of transfused children (compared with adults) experience transfusion reactions.[3–6] Despite data showing a decrease in blood transfusions across the United States in adults,[2,7] the 2017 National Blood Collection and Utilization Survey (NBCUS) showed a 7% to 14% increase in the

[a] Department of Laboratory Medicine, Yale University, New Haven, CT, USA; [b] Department of Pediatrics, Yale University, New Haven, CT, USA
* Corresponding author. 330 Cedar Street, CB 405, New Haven, CT 06520-8035.
E-mail address: jeanne.hendrickson@yale.edu

Clin Lab Med 41 (2021) 51–67
https://doi.org/10.1016/j.cll.2020.10.004
0272-2712/21/© 2020 Elsevier Inc. All rights reserved.

number of red blood cell (RBC), platelet, and plasma units transfused in neonates and children compared with 2015 using matched facility data.[2] As such, the total number of transfusion reactions in children would be expected to increase accordingly. This article reviews what is known about transfusion reactions in neonates and children, with a focus on definitions, pathophysiology, statistics, and mitigation strategies for the most common reactions.

HEMOVIGILANCE SYSTEMS

According to The International Hemovigilance Network (IHN) Web site,[8] the word hemovigilance means "a set of surveillance procedures covering the whole transfusion chain (from the collection of blood and its components to the follow-up of recipients), intended to collect and assess information on unexpected or undesirable effects resulting from the therapeutic use of labile blood products, and to prevent their occurrence or recurrence." Hemovigilance exists on local, national, and international levels, with groups from multiple countries having made extremely significant contributions over the past few decades.[9] The United Kingdom's Serious Hazards of Transfusion (UK-SHOT) reporting system[10] is one such notable example. The United States system is voluntary and relies on passive reporting using the Hemovigilance Module of the National Healthcare Safety Network (NHSN), initiated in 2009 to 2010.[11]

Although some hemovigilance systems (such as UK-SHOT) evaluate pediatric-specific data, systems in many other countries do not. Reporting systems' inconsistencies in combination with variability in reporting practices (ie, passive vs active), in addition to the retrospective nature of most studies, make studying trends in serious hazards of transfusion experienced by pediatric patients difficult. For example, as a part of the National Heart, Lung, and Blood Institute REDS-III (Recipient Epidemiology and Donor Evaluation Study) multicenter study, each participating US hospital identified significant underreporting in passive systems in adult transfusion recipients: fewer than 10% of pulmonary transfusion reactions identified by the clinical teams were reported to the transfusion service.[12]

ACUTE TRANSFUSION REACTIONS
Allergic Transfusion Reactions

Allergic transfusion reactions are reviewed first, because they are the most common type to be reported in children. Symptoms may range from mild urticaria and flushing to severe angioedema and bronchospasm/respiratory distress, occurring within 4 hours of the cessation of the transfusion.[13] Plasma proteins in the blood component are often implicated in such reactions, although transfusion recipient characteristics also likely contribute.[14,15]

A direct comparison of transfusion reaction rates in children and adults at a single tertiary care institution in the United States was published by Oakley and colleagues[5] in 2015. Over the 2-year study period, the incidence of allergic transfusion reactions in children was 2.7 per 1000, compared with 1.1 per 1000 in adults. Another study evaluated composite data from multiple pediatric and adult US hospitals over a 7-year study period and reported the incidence of allergic transfusion reactions in children to be 3.23 per 1000, compared with 0.72 per 1000 in adults[4] (**Fig. 1**). After breaking allergic reactions out by component type, the largest difference (7-fold) between children and adults occurred following RBC transfusion (2.78 per 1000 in children compared with 0.37 per 1000 in adults) and the next largest difference (3-fold) between children and adults was following platelet transfusion (6.24 per 1000 in children and 1.83 per 1000 in adults)[4] (**Fig. 2**). Studies outside the United States have also

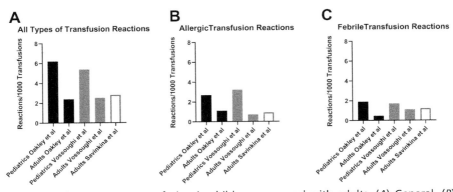

Fig. 1. Reaction rates per transfusion in children compared with adults. (*A*) General, (*B*) allergic, and (*C*) febrile nonhemolytic transfusion reaction rates in children compared with adults, as published by Oakley and colleagues[5] and Vossoughi and colleagues,[4] and in adults by the 2015 to 2017 National Blood Collection and Utilization Survey as published by Savinkina and colleagues.[114]

reported allergic reactions to be prevalent in children. For example, Pedrosa and colleagues[16] reported that 77% of transfusion reactions that occurred in children in Brazil were allergic and most commonly associated with platelets. Yanagisawa and colleagues[17] reported that allergic transfusion reactions were 4-fold more common than febrile nonhemolytic transfusion reactions in children studied in Japan, with platelets also being the blood component most frequently implicated. Li and colleagues[18] found that few identified allergic transfusion reactions to platelets were

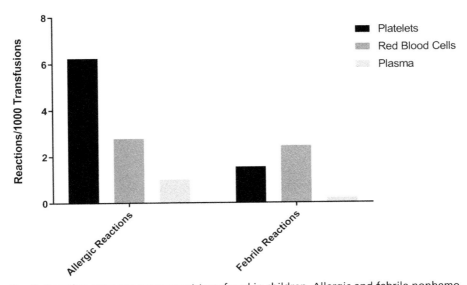

Fig. 2. Reaction rates per component transfused in children. Allergic and febrile nonhemolytic reaction rates in pediatric patients after transfusion of platelets, RBCs, or plasma; data by Vossoughi and colleagues.[4]

reported to the blood bank in a single-institution study, with all such reactions occurring in patients with hematologic or oncologic diseases. Moncharmont and Meyer[19] reported half of the reactions identified in pediatric patients to be allergic, with cutaneous being the most common manifestation. The 2018 UK-SHOT Annual Report found that allergic reactions to platelets were the most common reaction in the febrile/allergic/hypotensive category to occur in children, with most reactions occurring in the age group 1 to 16 years old.[20]

Few studies have separately evaluated anaphylactic transfusion reactions from less severe allergic transfusion reactions in children. Notably, the 2018 UK-SHOT Annual Report categorized 10 of the reported 26 allergic or mixed allergic/febrile reactions in children to be severe, including anaphylactic: 8 after platelet transfusion and 2 after plasma transfusion.[20] Immunoglobulin A (IgA) deficiency or the congenital absence of haptoglobin, responsible for some anaphylactic transfusion reactions,[21–23] may be diagnosed in a child for the first time following blood product exposure. The time range between transfusion initiation and symptoms of anaphylaxis is broad, although such severe reactions may occur in closer proximity to the initiation of the transfusion compared with milder allergic reactions.[17]

One reason that has been put forward to explain differences in allergic transfusion reaction rates between children and adults is the increased attentiveness and reporting of such symptoms in pediatric patients.[24] Vossoughi and colleagues[24] found that, in the setting of use of similar passive reporting systems, pediatric providers reported more reactions determined to be attributable to the transfusion than adult providers. The contribution of the issue of increased attention paid to symptoms in children resulting in higher allergic transfusion rates in this patient population is difficult to measure.

With the knowledge that children are more prone to allergic transfusion reactions than adults, are there any prophylactic measures to enact? Premedication with antihistamines (H1 or H2 blockers) has not been shown to decrease allergic transfusion reaction rates in children that have not previously had such reactions.[25,26] However, 1 recent study of children and adolescents with thalassemia did find that premedication might be beneficial in prevention of delayed urticaria.[27] From a component perspective, because the role of plasma proteins in allergic reactions is established, apheresis platelets stored in platelet additive solution have been reported to be associated with lower allergic transfusion reaction rates compared with apheresis platelets stored in plasma.[28,29] Also, solvent-detergent–treated plasma is associated with fewer allergic reactions compared with untreated plasma.[30] Washing blood components to decrease plasma content can also reduce allergic transfusion reactions, at a cost of decreased shelf life and product loss/damage caused by additional product manipulation.[31] Malvik and colleagues[32] recently described a 2-fold lower risk of allergic transfusion reactions following the transfusion of ABO-compatible platelets compared with major ABO-incompatible platelets. Provision of components from IgA-deficient donors or the selection of washed components is recommended for IgA-deficient recipients with detectable anti-IgA antibody levels.[33]

Febrile Nonhemolytic Transfusion Reactions

Ranking second in incidence behind allergic reactions are febrile nonhemolytic transfusion reactions (FNHTRs) (see Fig. 1). These reactions are defined by the US Centers for Disease Control and Prevention (CDC) as a patient's increase of body temperature to 38°C or more and a change of at least 1°C above baseline, or chills/rigors, occurring within 4 hours of the cessation of a transfusion.[13] Cytokines from residual white blood cells or recipient antibodies to donor antigens are thought to be responsible for

FNHTR. Fever may occur and has multiple causes; therefore, FNHTR is a diagnosis of exclusion. Underlying disease, hemolytic transfusion reaction, septic transfusion reaction, or transfusion-related acute lung injury (TRALI) should be considered in the differential diagnosis of a patient presenting with such a fever in temporal association with a transfusion.

Over the 2-year study period, the incidence of FNHTR in children studied by Oakley and colleagues[5] was 1.9 per 1000, compared with 0.47 per 1000 in adults; reaction rates were also noted to be significantly higher in male children (2.62 reactions per 100 males) compared with female children (1.2 reactions per 100 females). The study evaluated composite data from multiple pediatric and adult hospitals over a 7-year study period and also reported a higher incidence of FNHTR in children (1.71 per 1000) compared with in adults (1.1 per 1000)[4]; this study reported RBCs (2.46 per 1000) to be more likely to be associated with FNHTR compared with platelets (1.55 per 1000) or other products. Like Oakley and colleagues[5] and Vossoughi and colleagues,[24] Yanagisawa and colleagues[17] also reported FNHTR to be second in incidence behind allergic reactions in their studied pediatric cohort. This study also found that FNHTRs were more likely to occur in association with RBC transfusions, and found that males were 2.6-fold more likely to experience such reactions compared with females. Of note, the 2018 UK-SHOT Annual Report found only 4 per 30 reactions in the pediatric febrile/allergic/hypotensive category to be solely febrile.[20]

Fever occurring around the time of transfusion leads to considerable downstream costs, which have recently been quantitated.[34] Thus, measures to decrease such reactions are of significant interest. Premedication with antipyretics has not been shown to decrease the incidence of FNHTR,[35] although it may allow the completion of transfusions in patients with preexisting fever.[36] As mentioned earlier, because of the role of residual white blood cell cytokines in RBC products, FNHTRs are approximately 50% less likely to occur with the use of prestorage leukoreduced RBCs compared with non-leukoreduced components.[37] In addition to being associated with a lower incidence of allergic transfusion reactions, platelets stored in platelet additive solutions are also associated with a lower incidence of FNHTR.[28] Malvik and colleagues[32] recently described a 3-fold lower rate of FNHTR in children and adults transfused with ABO-identical platelets compared with those transfused with major ABO-mismatched platelets; these findings suggest that the A/B antigens in the platelet product complexing with recipient isohemagglutinins also may play a role.

Pulmonary Transfusion Reactions

Pulmonary complications from transfusions range from transfusion-associated dyspnea (TAD) to transfusion-associated circulatory overload (TACO) and TRALI. These reactions are each defined slightly differently depending on the reference source; the pathophysiology of TACO and TRALI has recently been extensively reviewed by Semple and colleagues.[38]

Pulmonary transfusion reactions in children may be less common compared with such reactions in adults, although few studies have investigated this topic in detail. Oakley and colleagues[5] reported 0.17 per 1000 cases of TACO in children (many <1 year old), which was not significantly different compared with the rate of 0.23 per 1000 reported in adults. Vossoughi and colleagues[4] reported 0.05 per 1000 cases of TAD, 0.03 per 1000 cases of TACO, and 0.02 per 1000 cases of TRALI in children. The 2018 UK-SHOT Annual Report described 4 cases of TACO, 2 caused by overtransfusion.[20] In contrast, after a detailed chart review, Li and colleagues[18] identified multiple cases of TAD, composing 45% of all identified acute transfusion reactions. Very few of the reactions identified by Li and colleagues[18] were reported to the transfusion service, a finding consistent with the very low reporting rate of pulmonary transfusion reactions in adults in 1 multihospital study. A Canadian retrospective case review of TRALI in children from 2001 to 2011 reported an incidence rate of 0.06 per 1000 RBC transfusions, compared with 0.04 per 1000 RBC transfusions in adults[39]; RBCs were the implicated product in more than half of the pediatric cases and some cases occurred in neonates. LaGrandeur and colleagues[40] also reported a case of TRALI in an infant following ligation of a patent ductus arteriosis, and Gupta and colleagues[41] reported TRALI in an infant as well. In a retrospective analysis, Thalji and colleagues[42] reported some type of pulmonary transfusion complication in 3.6% of pediatric surgery patients, with RBCs being the component most often implicated.

Note that most transfusion reaction definitions, including those of pulmonary reactions, were created based on data collected predominantly from adults. A 2018 study of pulmonary symptoms in pediatric patients in the intensive care unit by De Cloedt and colleagues,[43] highlights the importance of the diagnostic criteria; the investigators identified significantly different incidence rates of TACO in studied patients depending on the criteria used. To investigate whether respiratory decompensation occurred around the time of transfusion (to an extent that may not meet classic transfusion reaction definitions), another study closely evaluated respiratory status in extremely low birth weight neonates in periods after transfusion or in control time periods; the investigators reported no differences in acute respiratory decompensation between the 2 periods.[44]

Strategies to minimize pulmonary transfusion reactions in children and neonates are similar to those used in adults. Attention to blood volumes and ordered transfusion volumes is recommended, because the transfused product volume per blood volume is typically significantly higher at baseline in neonates and children than in adults. For example, 15 mL/kg of RBCs ordered for a 4-kg neonate whose blood volume is 90 mL/kg is a much higher proportion (60 mL/360 mL = 17%) compared with a 300-mL unit of RBCs ordered for a 90-kg adult whose blood volume is 70 mL/kg (300 mL/6300 mL = 4.8%). The 2018 UK-SHOT Annual Report found a disproportionate number of pediatric cases in the avoidable, delayed, or undertransfusion or overtransfusion category.[20]

Hypotensive Transfusion Reactions

Hypotensive transfusion reactions are defined by the CDC in children as a 25% decrease in systolic blood pressure occurring within 1 hour of the cessation of the transfusion in the absence of another explanation.[13] The cause of hypotensive transfusion reactions is not well understood, and thus the primary mitigation strategy is judicious transfusion. Bradykinins and their metabolites are thought to play a prominent role, leading to vasodilation. Hypotensive transfusion reactions have been described in patients taking angiotensin-converting enzyme inhibitors, with altered bradykinin breakdown being thought to be responsible.[45,46] However, hypotensive transfusion reactions also occur in patients not taking these drugs, and it has also been proposed that polymorphisms in aminopeptidase P or other enzymes that play a role in bradykinin breakdown may be in part responsible for this type of transfusion reaction.[47] A study conducted by Du Pont-Thibodeau and colleagues[48] failed to find a correlation between bradykinin levels in platelet concentrates and hypotensive transfusion reactions.

Hypotensive transfusion reactions may be more common in children than in adults. Oakley and colleagues[5] reported 0.29 per 1000 such reactions in children, compared with 0.078 per 1000 reactions in adults. Vossoughi and colleagues[4] reported a rate of 0.05 per 1000 in children, compared with 0.04 per 1000 in adults. In a chart review by

Li and colleagues,[18] 6.7% of the reactions identified (in 8/805 = 1% of studied platelet transfusions) were hypotensive. In 2006, Gauvin and colleagues[6] reported 3 severe hypotensive reactions to transfused platelets in children in the intensive care unit, out of 2509 total transfusions (0.12% of all transfusions).

Acute Hemolytic Transfusion Reactions

Acute hemolytic transfusion reactions (AHTRs) may be immune mediated (ABO related or non–ABO related) or non–immune mediated (primarily caused by mechanical hemolysis). Immune-mediated hemolysis is described in more detail here, although non–immune-mediated hemolysis should also be in the differential diagnosis, especially following transfusion through a small-gauge needle, following transfusion through a malfunctioning blood warmer, or following coadministration of RBCs with an incompatible type of intravenous solution. AHTRs may manifest with fever or chills, either alone,[36] or in combination with back/flank pain, pain at the intravenous access site, or several other symptoms.[49]

Attention has been paid to the role that isohemagglutinins in plasma-containing platelet products may play in AHTRs, in adults and in children.[50] Multiple cases of hemolysis caused by passively transferred anti-A have been described,[51,52] with anti-B being less likely to be reported to cause hemolysis.[53] Prior publications and review articles have discussed what a safe isohemagglutinin titer may be,[52–56] with this topic being of increasing interest as low-titer group O whole blood is being more widely used across the United States.

AHTRs caused by transfused RBCs most often occur in mistransfusion situations,[57] with errors in the transfusion process accounting for more than 60% of all reports to the UK-SHOT in the pediatric category and an even higher percentage in the neonatal/infant group.[58,59] Mistransfusion may occur primarily because of sample misidentification (eg, wrong blood in tube), although patient misidentification may also be responsible.[60] There have been situations described in which young siblings were mistaken for each other, or in which samples drawn from neonates were mistaken for samples drawn from their mothers.[58] Multiple strategies are in place in hospitals and clinics to prevent such mistransfusions from occurring, ranging from sample collection to blood bank testing to verification at the transfusion step. Some neonatal intensive care units provide group O RBCs to all patients regardless of ABO type, to decrease the likelihood of a mistransfusion situation. However, the short-term and longer-term consequences of the out-of-group plasma contained in the group O RBCs remains to be determined.[61] In addition to ABO incompatibility, AHTRs may also (albeit rarely) occur because of recipient non-ABO alloantibodies in instances of mistransfusion.

Few data exist to compare the rate of AHTRs in children with that in adults. Oakley and colleagues[5] did not identify any AHTRs in the studied pediatric population. Vossoughi and colleagues[4] reported 10 times more AHTRs caused by RBCs in children (0.09 per 1000) than in adults (0.009 per 1000), with no differences in the rate of these reactions caused by platelets and no AHTRs reported in association with other blood components.

DELAYED TRANSFUSION REACTIONS
Alloantibody Induction

RBC transfusion may lead to alloantibody induction to non-ABO blood group antigens in some transfusion recipients, particularly those with sickle cell disease or thalassemia.[62] Patients with myelodysplastic syndromes[63] and patients with autoimmune disease[64] are also more likely to form RBC alloantibodies after transfusion compared with other patient populations. According to some reports, RBC alloimmunization is the most common delayed transfusion reaction. Alloimmunization prevalence rates increase with age, given increasing exposure history through transfusion as well as through pregnancy. As a generalization, alloantibodies are unlikely to form before the age of 1 year,[65] although case reports describe antibody formation in younger infants.[66,67]

In addition to leading to delays in locating compatible RBC units for subsequent transfusions, RBC alloantibodies increase the risk for acute or delayed hemolytic transfusion reactions and, in females, introduce a risk of hemolytic disease of the fetus and newborn. The primary strategy to prevent alloimmunization is transfusion or pregnancy avoidance. When transfusion is necessary, the provision of RBCs phenotypically matched for some of the most immunogenic antigens (C/c, E/e, and K) is recommended for patients with sickle cell disease[68] and with thalassemia[69] to decrease the likelihood of alloantibody formation. In patients with existing alloantibodies, extending the degree of antigen matching for antigens such as Fy, Jk, and S may be beneficial when feasible.[69] Given antibody evanescence in combination with often fragmented health care patterns,[70] it is important that patients and their parents are aware of all antibodies and their potential future implications.

Besides antigens on RBCs, alloantibodies to human leukocyte antigens (HLAs) can also be induced. Multiple studies have found a correlation between RBC alloantibodies and HLA alloantibodies, including studies completed in children with sickle cell disease in which leukoreduced RBCs were the only known exposure trigger.[71–73] Resultant HLA antibodies may lead to platelet transfusion refractoriness and may also be significant in solid organ or hematopoietic stem cell transplant settings.[74,75]

Delayed Serologic and Delayed Hemolytic Transfusion Reaction

Delayed serologic transfusion reactions (DSTRs) and delayed hemolytic transfusion reactions (DHTRs) occur in children as well as in adults. DSTRs are significantly more common than DHTRs,[76,77] occurring when an antibody is detected by the transfusion service between 24 hours and 28 days posttransfusion and not resulting in noticeable hemolysis.[13,49] In contrast, DHTRs result in an inadequate increase or a rapid decrease of hemoglobin level in the setting of a newly identified antibody[49] (ie, the antibody in question is typically present below the level of detection at the time of the transfusion, having evanesced at some point in the past). More than 60% to 70% of antibodies, including those of most specificities, evanesce over time in patients[78] as well as in healthy blood donors.[79]

Reporting data on DSTRs/DHTRs vary between countries and between studies, and a few studies have compared DSTR or DHTR rates in children with those in adults. Oakley and colleagues[5] found no DSTRs and 1 DHTR in children compared with 8 DSTRs and 3 DHTRs in adults. Vossoughi and colleagues[4] found 1 DHTR in children (0.0075 per 1000) compared with 36 (0.065 per 1000) in adults. The incidence of DHTR in patients with sickle cell disease is high compared with other transfusion reactions, ranging from 2.2% to 9% per patient.[80] This rate is likely to be underestimated, because DHTRs in this population may be misdiagnosed as vaso-occlusive episodes.

DHTRs with bystander hemolysis (also referred to as hyperhemolysis) involve destruction not only of transfused RBCs but also of the patient's own RBCs. Such reactions can be particularly severe in patients with sickle cell disease,[81–83] and the mortality secondary to RBC alloimmunization/DHTRs is greater than previously appreciated.[84,85] Approximately half of all DHTRs with bystander hemolysis are associated with newly detectable RBC alloantibodies, although many occur in patients with a history of RBC alloimmunization.[76] Treatment of such reactions may involve transfusion avoidance, administration of erythropoietin, supplemental iron, immunosuppression, and, if life threatening, complement inhibition.[68]

The primary prevention of DSTRs, DHTRs, and antibody-associated DHTRs with bystander hemolysis is judicious transfusion in combination with a centralized antibody registry accessible across hospitals and health care systems. With such a registry,[86] previously detected antibodies that have become evanescent will be known and thus antigen-negative RBC units can be selected to increase transfusion safety.

Transfusion-Associated Graft-Versus-Host Disease

Transfusion-associated graft-versus-host disease (TA-GVHD) is a rare but often deadly complication that occurs 2 days to 6 weeks after a transfusion into at-risk individuals. Mediated by donor lymphocytes, at-risk recipients include those that are immunocompromised or receiving blood components from genetically similar individuals.[36] Fetuses requiring intrauterine transfusions are at risk of TA-GVHD, as are neonates receiving exchange transfusions and those with potentially undiagnosed immunodeficiencies.[87] Among others, children undergoing stem cell transplant, treatment with chemotherapy, or receiving crossmatched/HLA-matched platelets are also at risk.[87] Although TA-GVHD is associated with high mortality in adults, there have been few reported cases in fetuses, neonates, or children.[88]

Strategies to mitigate the risk of TA-GVHD are based on inactivation of white cells in cellular products by irradiation or treatment with pathogen reduction technologies.[89] Some hospitals irradiate blood products for neonates below a certain age to decrease the likelihood of missing an undiagnosed immunodeficiency, whereas others irradiate at the request of the treating physician. Some clinicians have argued for universal/default irradiation policies at hospitals caring for children, given the high stakes of missed irradiation events in combination with errors that occur when blood banks rely on providers to order the correct blood product modification for at-risk transfusion recipients.[87]

Transfusion-Transmitted Infections

In the authors' experience, transfusion-transmitted viral infections are the leading concern of parents as they sign consent for their children to receive a blood product. However, such infections are many logs less likely to occur than most of the other adverse transfusion reactions reviewed in this article. Consenting providers should be well versed in the current testing requirements as well as the current infectious disease transmission risks, which are described in detail by Busch and colleagues.[90] At present in the United States, the risk of transfusion-transmitted hepatitis B, hepatitis C, or human immunodeficiency virus is approximately 1 in 2 million and the risk of transfusion-transmitted human T-lymphotropic virus-1/II is approximately 1 in 3 million. The risk of other transfusion-transmitted viral infections is also low, with estimates for Zika virus, West Nile virus, and cytomegalovirus being less than 1 in 3 million.[90] Given these low numbers, very few cases of transfusion-transmitted viral infections have been reported in neonates or children in the modern era.[88]

Transfusion-transmitted bacterial infections are significantly more likely to occur than transfusion-transmitted viral infections, with bacterial contamination risk for platelets on the day of transfusion estimated to be 1 in 2500.[91] Strategies on the blood collection, manufacturing, and testing sides (including pathogen reduction technology[92]) are increasingly being incorporated across the globe to mitigate such risk. Real-world experience with pathogen-reduced platelets is currently being accumulated in the United States, with no unexpected nonimmunologic adverse events observed following pathogen-reduced platelet transfusion in adult or pediatric patients at the authors' institution.[93,94] However, at the same institution, there was a significant temporal increase in platelet transfusions and immune-mediated platelet transfusion refractoriness in adults as well as in children following the introduction of pathogen-reduced platelets[95]; it remains unclear whether the observations are causal. As recommendations in the 2019 US Food and Drug Administration guidance ("Bacterial Risk Control Strategies for Blood Collection Establishments and Transfusion Services to Enhance the Safety and Availability of Platelets for Transfusion")[96] are put into place, the risk of transfusion-transmitted bacterial infections in platelets is predicted to decline.

Transfusion-transmitted parasitic infections are rare but do occur in children. For example, at the authors' institution, there was a cluster of 3 cases of transfusion-transmitted babesiosis in neonates traced to a single contaminated donor unit.[97] Hospital RBC allocation practices affect the number of neonates potentially exposed to such infected units.

OTHER

There are other posttransfusion sequelae in neonates and children. Iron overload is one of the well-known and studied complications of repeated RBC transfusions,[98] occurring in children and neonates.[88] It can lead to cardiac, hepatic, and endocrine complications, particularly in children with thalassemia or sickle cell disease undergoing chronic RBC transfusion therapy. Iron chelation therapies, reviewed by Kwiatkowski,[99] are the primary strategies for transfusion-dependent patients with thalassemia; iron load can be better controlled in patients with sickle cell disease through the use of RBC exchange (rather than simple) transfusions. Attention has also recently been paid to the iron burden that children with malignancies accumulate following supportive-care RBC transfusions.[100,101]

Electrolyte/metabolic complications may be more likely to occur following transfusion in neonates or children than in adults, because of size/volume considerations in combination with the immature liver of neonates. Hypocalcemia caused by citrate exposure has been most studied in adult massive transfusion situations[102] and may also occur in neonates following exchange transfusions. Hypoglycemia may also occur following neonatal exchange transfusions if fluids containing dextrose are discontinued. Hyperkalemia severe enough to result in cardiac arrest has been reported following massive, rapid infusion of RBCs in neonates and children.[103] In contrast, single aliquots (<20 mL/kg) of RBCs transfused over the typical 2 to 4 hours are unlikely to lead to harm.[104]

In addition, there are clinical outcomes in neonates that are not considered classic transfusion reactions per se but that are worth mentioning. Association data exist between RBC transfusion and necrotizing enterocolitis (NEC).[88,105] Patel and colleagues[110] have published that the severity of underlying anemia at the time of the transfusion plays a more critical role in developing NEC than the transfusion itself,[106,107] a conclusion supported by animal model data.[108] Other than NEC, questions regarding possible associations between RBC or platelet transfusions and outcomes such as bronchopulmonary dysplasia/chronic lung disease, retinopathy of prematurity, and intraventricular hemorrhage have been raised.[59,109]

COMPONENT MODIFICATIONS AND STORAGE DURATION

Reviewed in more depth in other articles in this series, blood component modifications and storage duration are worth briefly mentioning in the context of adverse transfusion reactions. Increasing irradiation storage duration has been shown to be associated with metabolomic RBC changes[110] and increased risk of nonallergic transfusion reactions.[111] In contrast, RBC storage duration in general has not been found to affect studied outcomes in neonatal[112] or pediatric populations.[113]

SUMMARY

Transfusion reaction types and incidence are different in neonates and children compared with those in adults. Although some reactions (particularly allergic) are more common in the pediatric population, transfusion reactions have been better studied in adults. The recently published Randomized Trial of Platelet-Transfusion Thresholds in Neonates (PlaNeT2) study[109] has opened a dialogue surrounding complications potentially associated with transfusions are not covered by the classic transfusion reaction definitions. There is an ongoing need for robust hemovigilance systems, such that accurate data can be collected. Further, increased attention needs to be paid to pediatric transfusion reactions, to understand pathophysiologic differences that may account for the higher transfusion reaction rates in this population and to develop strategies to decrease such reactions.

DISCLOSURE

The authors have nothing to disclose.

REFERENCES

1. Morley SL, Hudson CL, Llewelyn CA, et al. Transfusion in children: epidemiology and 10-year survival of transfusion recipients. Transfus Med 2016;26(2):111–7.
2. Sapiano MRP, Jones JM, Savinkina AA, et al. Supplemental findings of the 2017 National blood collection and utilization survey. Transfusion 2020;60(Suppl 2): S17–37.
3. Lavoie J. Blood transfusion risks and alternative strategies in pediatric patients. Paediatr Anaesth 2011;21(1):14–24.
4. Vossoughi S, Perez G, Whitaker BI, et al. Analysis of pediatric adverse reactions to transfusions. Transfusion 2018;58(1):60–9.
5. Oakley FD, Woods M, Arnold S, et al. Transfusion reactions in pediatric compared with adult patients: a look at rate, reaction type, and associated products. Transfusion 2015;55(3):563–70.
6. Gauvin F, Lacroix J, Robillard P, et al. Acute transfusion reactions in the pediatric intensive care unit. Transfusion 2006;46(11):1899–908.
7. Jones JM, Sapiano MRP, Savinkina AA, et al. Slowing decline in blood collection and transfusion in the United States - 2017. Transfusion 2020;60(Suppl 2):S1–9.
8. International Haemovigilance Network. Available at: www.ihn-org.com. Accessed February 15, 2020.
9. Wood EM, Ang AL, Bisht A, et al. International haemovigilance: what have we learned and what do we need to do next? Transfus Med 2019;29(4):221–30.
10. Bolton-Maggs PHB. Conference report: international haemovigilance seminar and the SHOT annual symposium, 10-12 july 2018. Transfus Med 2019;29(4): 247–52.
11. Chung KW, Harvey A, Basavaraju SV, et al. How is national recipient hemovigilance conducted in the United States? Transfusion 2015;55(4):703–7.
12. Hendrickson JE, Roubinian NH, Chowdhury D, et al. Incidence of transfusion reactions: a multicenter study utilizing systematic active surveillance and expert adjudication. Transfusion 2016;56(10):2587–96.

13. NHSN biovigilance component: hemovigilance Module surveillance protocol v2.5.2. 2018. Available at: www.cdc.gov/nhsn. Accesssed February 15, 2020.

14. Savage WJ, Hamilton RG, Tobian AA, et al. Defining risk factors and presentations of allergic reactions to platelet transfusion. J Allergy Clin Immunol 2014; 133(6):1772–5.e9.

15. Savage WJ, Tobian AA, Savage JH, et al. Transfusion and component characteristics are not associated with allergic transfusion reactions to apheresis platelets. Transfusion 2015;55(2):296–300.

16. Pedrosa AK, Pinto FJ, Lins LD, et al. Blood transfusion reactions in children: associated factors. J Pediatr (Rio J) 2013;89(4):400–6.

17. Yanagisawa R, Tatsuzawa Y, Ono T, et al. Analysis of clinical presentations of allergic transfusion reactions and febrile non-haemolytic transfusion reactions in paediatric patients. Vox Sang 2019;114(8):826–34.

18. Li N, Williams L, Zhou Z, et al. Incidence of acute transfusion reactions to platelets in hospitalized pediatric patients based on the US hemovigilance reporting system. Transfusion 2014;54(6):1666–72.

19. Moncharmont P, Meyer F. [Allergic adverse transfusion reactions in paediatrics, a 3-year study]. Transfus Clin Biol 2013;20(5–6):455–7.

20. S. Narayan (Ed), E. Poles, et al, on behalf of the Serious Hazards of Transfusion (SHOT) Steering Group. The 2018 Annual Report (2019). Available at: https://www.shotuk.org/wp-content/uploads/myimages/SHOTReport-2018_Web_Version.pdf. Accessed 15 February, 2020.

21. Ando J, Masuda A, Iizuka K, et al. Congenital haptoglobin deficiency discovered on the occasion of anaphylaxis induced by platelet concentrate transfusion. Rinsho Ketsueki 2016;57(12):2507–11.

22. Sandler SG, Eder AF, Goldman M, et al. The entity of immunoglobulin A-related anaphylactic transfusion reactions is not evidence based. Transfusion 2015; 55(1):199–204.

23. Thoren KL, Avecilla ST, Klimek V, et al. A novel method for the laboratory workup of anaphylactic transfusion reactions in haptoglobin-deficient patients. Transfusion 2020;60(4):682–7.

24. Vossoughi S, Parker-Jones S, Schwartz J, et al. Provider trends in paediatric and adult transfusion reaction reporting. Vox Sang 2019;114(3):232–6.

25. Duran J, Siddique S, Cleary M. Effects of leukoreduction and premedication with acetaminophen and diphenhydramine in minimizing febrile nonhemolytic transfusion reactions and allergic transfusion reactions during and after blood product administration: a literature review with recommendations for practice. J Pediatr Oncol Nurs 2014;31(4):223–9.

26. Sanders RP, Maddirala SD, Geiger TL, et al. Premedication with acetaminophen or diphenhydramine for transfusion with leucoreduced blood products in children. Br J Haematol 2005;130(5):781–7.

27. Rujkijyanont P, Monsereenusorn C, Manoonphol P, et al. Efficacy of oral acetaminophen and intravenous chlorpheniramine maleate versus placebo to prevent red cell transfusion reactions in children and adolescent with thalassemia: a prospective, randomized, double-blind controlled trial. Anemia 2018;2018:9492303.

28. van Hout FMA, van der Meer PF, Wiersum-Osselton JC, et al. Transfusion reactions after transfusion of platelets stored in PAS-B, PAS-C, or plasma: a nationwide comparison. Transfusion 2018;58(4):1021–7.

29. Pagano MB, Katchatag BL, Khoobyari S, et al. Evaluating safety and cost-effectiveness of platelets stored in additive solution (PAS-F) as a hemolysis risk mitigation strategy. Transfusion 2019;59(4):1246–51.

30. Saadah NH, van der Bom JG, Wiersum-Osselton JC, et al. Comparing transfusion reaction risks for various plasma products - an analysis of 7 years of IS-TARE haemovigilance data. Br J Haematol 2018;180(5):727–34.

31. Karafin M, Fuller AK, Savage WJ, et al. The impact of apheresis platelet manipulation on corrected count increment. Transfusion 2012;52(6):1221–7.

32. Malvik N, Leon J, Schlueter AJ, et al. ABO-incompatible platelets are associated with increased transfusion reaction rates. Transfusion 2020;60(2):285–93.

33. Simons FE, Ebisawa M, Sanchez-Borges M, et al. 2015 update of the evidence base: World Allergy Organization anaphylaxis guidelines. World Allergy Organ J 2015;8(1):32.

34. Cohen R, Escorcia A, Tasmin F, et al. Feeling the burn: the significant burden of febrile nonhemolytic transfusion reactions. Transfusion 2017;57(7):1674–83.

35. Kennedy LD, Case LD, Hurd DD, et al. A prospective, randomized, double-blind controlled trial of acetaminophen and diphenhydramine pretransfusion medication versus placebo for the prevention of transfusion reactions. Transfusion 2008;48(11):2285–91.

36. Delaney M, Wendel S, Bercovitz RS, et al. Transfusion reactions: prevention, diagnosis, and treatment. Lancet 2016;388(10061):2825–36.

37. King KE, Shirey RS, Thoman SK, et al. Universal leukoreduction decreases the incidence of febrile nonhemolytic transfusion reactions to RBCs. Transfusion 2004;44(1):25–9.

38. Semple JW, Rebetz J, Kapur R. Transfusion-associated circulatory overload and transfusion-related acute lung injury. Blood 2019;133(17):1840–53.

39. Lieberman L, Petraszko T, Yi QL, et al. Transfusion-related lung injury in children: a case series and review of the literature. Transfusion 2014;54(1):57–64.

40. LaGrandeur RG, Tran M, Merchant C, et al. Transfusion-related acute lung injury following PDA ligation in a preterm neonate. J Neonatal Perinatal Med 2017; 10(3):339–42.

41. Gupta S, Som T, Iyer L, et al. Transfusion related acute lung injury in a neonate. Indian J Pediatr 2012;79(10):1363–5.

42. Thalji L, Thum D, Weister TJ, et al. Incidence and epidemiology of perioperative transfusion-related pulmonary complications in pediatric noncardiac surgical patients: a single-center, 5-year experience. Anesth Analg 2018;127(5):1180–8.

43. De Cloedt L, Emeriaud G, Lefebvre E, et al. Transfusion-associated circulatory overload in a pediatric intensive care unit: different incidences with different diagnostic criteria. Transfusion 2018;58(4):1037–44.

44. Grev JE, Stanclova M, Ellsworth MA, et al. Does red blood cell transfusion-related acute lung injury occur in premature infants? A retrospective cohort analysis. Am J Perinatol 2017;34(1):14–8.

45. Kalra A, Palaniswamy C, Patel R, et al. Acute hypotensive transfusion reaction with concomitant use of angiotensin-converting enzyme inhibitors: a case report and review of the literature. Am J Ther 2012;19(2):e90–4.

46. Doria C, Elia ES, Kang Y, et al. Acute hypotensive transfusion reaction during liver transplantation in a patient on angiotensin converting enzyme inhibitors from low aminopeptidase P activity. Liver Transpl 2008;14(5):684–7.

47. Hui Y, Wu Y, Tormey CA. The development of a novel molecular assay examining the role of aminopeptidase P polymorphisms in acute hypotensive transfusion reactions. Arch Pathol Lab Med 2013;137(1):96–9.

48. Du Pont-Thibodeau G, Robitaille N, Gauvin F, et al. Incidence of hypotension and acute hypotensive transfusion reactions following platelet concentrate transfusions. Vox Sang 2016;110(2):150–8.

49. Fabron A Jr, Moreira G Jr, Bordin JO. Delayed hemolytic transfusion reaction presenting as a painful crisis in a patient with sickle cell anemia. Sao Paulo Med J 1999;117(1):38–9.

50. Harris SB, Josephson CD, Kost CB, et al. Nonfatal intravascular hemolysis in a pediatric patient after transfusion of a platelet unit with high-titer anti-A. Transfusion 2007;47(8):1412–7.

51. Cooling L. ABO and platelet transfusion therapy. Immunohematology 2007; 23(1):20–33.

52. Josephson CD, Castillejo MI, Grima K, et al. ABO-mismatched platelet transfusions: strategies to mitigate patient exposure to naturally occurring hemolytic antibodies. Transfus Apher Sci 2010;42(1):83–8.

53. Balbuena-Merle R, West FB, Tormey CA, et al. Fatal acute hemolytic transfusion reaction due to anti-B from a platelet apheresis unit stored in platelet additive solution. Transfusion 2019;59(6):1911–5.

54. Dunbar NM, Katus MC, Freeman CM, et al. Easier said than done: ABO compatibility and D matching in apheresis platelet transfusions. Transfusion 2015;55(8): 1882–8.

55. Fontaine MJ, Webster J, Gomez S, et al. How do I implement an automated screen for high-titer ABO antibody as an inventory management tool for ABO plasma-incompatible platelets? Transfusion 2015;55(12):2783–9.

56. Berseus O, Boman K, Nessen SC, et al. Risks of hemolysis due to anti-A and anti-B caused by the transfusion of blood or blood components containing ABO-incompatible plasma. Transfusion 2013;53(Suppl 1):114S–23S.

57. Heddle NM, Fung M, Hervig T, et al. Challenges and opportunities to prevent transfusion errors: a qualitative evaluation for safer transfusion (QUEST). Transfusion 2012;52(8):1687–95.

58. Bolton-Maggs PH. Transfusion and hemovigilance in pediatrics. Pediatr Clin North Am 2013;60(6):1527–40.

59. Keir AK, New H, Robitaille N, et al. Approaches to understanding and interpreting the risks of red blood cell transfusion in neonates. Transfus Med 2019;29(4): 231–8.

60. Goel R, Tobian AAR, Shaz BH. Noninfectious transfusion-associated adverse events and their mitigation strategies. Blood 2019;133(17):1831–9.

61. Refaai MA, Cahill C, Masel D, et al. Is it time to reconsider the concepts of "universal donor" and "ABO compatible" transfusions? Anesth Analg 2018;126(6): 2135–8.

62. Tormey CA, Hendrickson JE. Transfusion-related red blood cell alloantibodies: induction and consequences. Blood 2019;133(17):1821–30.

63. Singhal D, Kutyna MM, Chhetri R, et al. Red cell alloimmunization is associated with development of autoantibodies and increased red cell transfusion requirements in myelodysplastic syndrome. Haematologica 2017;102(12):2021–9.

64. Karafin MS, Westlake M, Hauser RG, et al. Risk factors for red blood cell alloimmunization in the Recipient Epidemiology and Donor Evaluation Study (REDS-III) database. Br J Haematol 2018;181(5):672–81.

65. Turkmen T, Qiu D, Cooper N, et al. Red blood cell alloimmunization in neonates and children up to 3 years of age. Transfusion 2017;57(11):2720–6.

66. Tyler LN, Harville TO, Backall DP. Multiple alloantibodies after transfusion in an infant treated with Infliximab. N Engl J Med 2007;357:2092–3.

67. Hata JL, Johnson MS, Booth GS. Neonatal alloimmunization: a rare case of multiple alloantibody formation in a patient with disseminated histoplasmosis. Transfusion 2013;53(5):1140–1.

68. Chou ST, Alsawas M, Fasano RM, et al. American Society of Hematology 2020 guidelines for sickle cell disease: transfusion support. Blood Adv 2020;4(2): 327–55.

69. Trompeter S, Massey E, Robinson S. Position paper on International Collaboration for Transfusion Medicine (ICTM) Guideline 'Red blood cell specifications for patients with hemoglobinopathies: a systematic review and guideline'. Br J Haematol 2020;189(3):424–7.

70. Unni N, Peddinghaus M, Tormey CA, et al. Record fragmentation due to transfusion at multiple health care facilities: a risk factor for delayed hemolytic transfusion reactions. Transfusion 2014;54(1):98–103.

71. Nickel RS, Hendrickson JE, Yee MM, et al. Red blood cell transfusions are associated with HLA class I but not H-Y alloantibodies in children with sickle cell disease. Br J Haematol 2015;170(2):247–56.

72. Nickel RS, Horan JT, Fasano RM, et al. Immunophenotypic parameters and RBC alloimmunization in children with sickle cell disease on chronic transfusion. Am J Hematol 2015;90(12):1135–41.

73. McPherson ME, Anderson AR, Castillejo MI, et al. HLA alloimmunization is associated with RBC antibodies in multiply transfused patients with sickle cell disease. Pediatr Blood Cancer 2010;54(4):552–8.

74. Nickel RS, Horan JT, Abraham A, et al. Human leukocyte antigen (HLA) class I antibodies and transfusion support in paediatric HLA-matched haematopoietic cell transplant for sickle cell disease. Br J Haematol 2020;189(1):162–70.

75. Weinstock C, Schnaidt M. Human leucocyte antigen Sensitisation and its impact on transfusion practice. Transfus Med Hemother 2019;46(5):356–69.

76. Siddon AJ, Kenney BC, Hendrickson JE, et al. Delayed haemolytic and serologic transfusion reactions: pathophysiology, treatment and prevention. Curr Opin Hematol 2018;25(6):459–67.

77. Ness PM, Shirey RS, Thoman SK, et al. The differentiation of delayed serologic and delayed hemolytic transfusion reactions: incidence, long-term serologic findings, and clinical significance. Transfusion 1990;30(8):688–93.

78. Tormey CA, Stack G. The persistence and evanescence of blood group alloantibodies in men. Transfusion 2009;49(3):505–12.

79. Hauser RG, Esserman D, Karafin MS, et al. The evanescence and persistence of RBC alloantibodies in blood donors. Transfusion 2020;60(4):831–9.

80. Pirenne F, Yazdanbakhsh K. How I safely transfuse patients with sickle-cell disease and manage delayed hemolytic transfusion reactions. Blood 2018;131(25) 2773–81.

81. Gardner K, Hoppe C, Mijovic A, et al. How we treat delayed haemolytic transfusion reactions in patients with sickle cell disease. Br J Haematol 2015;170(6): 745–56.

82. Mekontso Dessap A, Pirenne F, Razazi K, et al. A diagnostic nomogram for delayed hemolytic transfusion reaction in sickle cell disease. Am J Hematol 2016; 91(12):1181–4.

83. Narbey D, Habibi A, Chadebech P, et al. Incidence and predictive score for delayed hemolytic transfusion reaction in adult patients with sickle cell disease. Am J Hematol 2017;92(12):1340–8.

84. Nickel RS, Hendrickson JE, Fasano RM, et al. Impact of red blood cell alloimmunization on sickle cell disease mortality: a case series. Transfusion 2016;56(1):107–14.

85. Thein SL, Pirenne F, Fasano RM, et al. Hemolytic transfusion reactions in sickle cell disease: underappreciated and potentially fatal. Haematologica 2020;105(3):539–44.

86. Hauser RG, Hendrickson JE, Tormey CA. TRIX with treats: the considerable safety benefits of a transfusion medicine registry. Transfusion 2019;59(8):2489–92.

87. Delaney M. How I reduce the risk of missed irradiation transfusion events in children. Transfusion 2018;58(11):2517–21.

88. Moncharmont P. Adverse transfusion reactions in transfused children. Transfus Clin Biol 2019;26(4):329–35.

89. Marschner S, Fast LD, Baldwin WM 3rd, et al. White blood cell inactivation after treatment with riboflavin and ultraviolet light. Transfusion 2010;50(11):2489–98.

90. Busch MP, Bloch EM, Kleinman S. Prevention of transfusion-transmitted infections. Blood 2019;133(17):1854–64.

91. Hong H, Xiao W, Lazarus HM, et al. Detection of septic transfusion reactions to platelet transfusions by active and passive surveillance. Blood 2016;127(4):496–502.

92. Devine DV. Implementation of pathogen inactivation technology: how to make the best decisions? Transfusion 2017;57(5):1109–11.

93. Bahar B, Schulz WL, Gokhale A, et al. Blood utilisation and transfusion reactions in adult patients transfused with conventional or pathogen-reduced platelets. Br J Haematol 2019;188(3):465–72.

94. Schulz WL, McPadden J, Gehrie EA, et al. Blood utilization and transfusion reactions in pediatric patients transfused with conventional or pathogen reduced platelets. J Pediatr 2019;209:220–5.

95. Hendrickson JE, Mendoza H, Ross R, et al. Investigation of increased platelet alloimmunization screening in the era of pathogen-reduced platelets treated with psoralen/UV light. Transfusion 2020;60(3):650–1.

96. US Dept of Health and Human Services. Bacterial risk control strategies for blood collection establishments and transfusion services to enhance the safety and availability of platelets for transfusion. Center for Biologics Evaluation and Research; 2019. Available at: https://www.fda.gov/vaccines-blood-biologics/guidance-compliance-regulatory-information-biologics/biologics-guidances. Accessed 15 February, 2020.

97. Glanternik JR, Baine IL, Rychalsky MR, et al. A cluster of cases of Babesia microti among neonates traced to a single unit of donor blood. Pediatr Infect Dis J 2018;37(3):269–71.

98. Coates TD. Iron overload in transfusion-dependent patients. Hematol Am Soc Hematol Educ Program 2019;2019(1):337–44.

99. Kwiatkowski JL. Current recommendations for chelation for transfusion-dependent thalassemia. Ann N Y Acad Sci 2016;1368(1):107–14.

100. Ruccione KS, Wood JC, Sposto R, et al. Characterization of transfusion-derived iron deposition in childhood cancer survivors. Cancer Epidemiol Biomarkers Prev 2014;23(9):1913–9.

101. Trovillion EM, Schubert L, Dietz AC. Iron overload in survivors of childhood cancer. J Pediatr Hematol Oncol 2018;40(5):396–400.

102. Ditzel RM Jr, Anderson JL, Eisenhart WJ, et al. A review of transfusion- and trauma-induced hypocalcemia. Is it time to change the lethal triad to the lethal diamond? J Trauma Acute Care Surg 2020;88(3):434–9.
103. Lee AC, Reduque LL, Luban NL, et al. Transfusion-associated hyperkalemic cardiac arrest in pediatric patients receiving massive transfusion. Transfusion 2014;54(1):244–54.
104. Strauss RG. RBC storage and avoiding hyperkalemia from transfusions to neonates & infants. Transfusion 2010;50(9):1862–5.
105. Maheshwari A, Patel RM, Christensen RD. Anemia, red blood cell transfusions, and necrotizing enterocolitis. Semin Pediatr Surg 2018;27(1):47–51.
106. Patel RM, Knezevic A, Shenvi N, et al. Association of red blood cell transfusion, anemia, and necrotizing enterocolitis in very low-birth-weight infants. JAMA 2016;315(9):889–97.
107. Saroha V, Josephson CD, Patel RM. Epidemiology of necrotizing enterocolitis: New considerations regarding the influence of red blood cell transfusions and anemia. Clin Perinatol 2019;46(1):101–17.
108. MohanKumar K, Namachivayam K, Song T, et al. A murine neonatal model of necrotizing enterocolitis caused by anemia and red blood cell transfusions. Nat Commun 2019;10(1):3494.
109. Curley A, Stanworth SJ, Willoughby K, et al. Randomized trial of platelet-transfusion thresholds in neonates. N Engl J Med 2019;380(3):242–51.
110. Patel RM, Roback JD, Uppal K, et al. Metabolomics profile comparisons of irradiated and nonirradiated stored donor red blood cells. Transfusion 2015;55(3): 544–52.
111. Chen J, Biller E, Losos M, et al. Irradiation and prolonged storage of red cells are associated with increased adverse events. Vox Sang 2018;113:468–75.
112. Fergusson DA, Hebert P, Hogan DL, et al. Effect of fresh red blood cell transfusions on clinical outcomes in premature, very low-birth-weight infants: the ARIPI randomized trial. JAMA 2012;308(14):1443–51.
113. Spinella PC, Tucci M, Fergusson DA, et al. Effect of fresh vs standard-issue red blood cell transfusions on multiple organ dysfunction syndrome in critically ill pediatric patients: a randomized clinical trial. JAMA 2019;322(22):2179–90.
114. Savinkina AA, Haass KA, Sapiano MRP, et al. Transfusion-associated adverse events and implementation of blood safety measures - findings from the 2017 National Blood Collection and Utilization Survey. Transfusion 2020;60(Suppl 2):S10–6.

Inventory Management and Product Selection in Pediatric Blood Banking

Jenna T. Reece, MD[a], Deborah Sesok-Pizzini, MD, MBA[b],*

KEYWORDS

- Inventory management • Blood use management • Blood wastage • Blood supply
- Manufacturing • Blood storage

KEY POINTS

- Inventory management in pediatric blood banking involves the balance between keeping an adequate supply of blood in the hospital for clinical care needs and reducing the wastage of expired products not transfused.
- Pediatric patients require special manufacturing of aliquots because of the smaller size of transfusions needed. These patients also require special considerations for freshness, leukocyte reduction, irradiation, and product selection compared with adult patients.
- Simple methods can be adopted to ensure that daily inventory is kept at the appropriate levels, and these steps involve close coordination with the blood bank and clinical teams as well as daily reconciliation of the inventory at hand with new orders and requests.

Inventory management for pediatric blood banking involves multiple manufacturing steps that ensure that the right product and the right volume is delivered to the patient at the right time. It is a complex process that involves comparison of blood issued with blood in inventory, making certain that units issued and units in storage are accounted for in the blood bank. Usually a manager or supervisor is responsible for this task and reviews daily reports and compares these reports with daily blood counts of stored inventory. As a result of these reconciliations, the blood bank staff know what amount of blood to order from their blood supplier to maintain average daily inventories. In most blood banks, pediatric and adult alike, there are minimum inventories established for each major ABO blood group (A+, A−, B+, B−, AB+, AB−, O+, O−) and for each available component type: red blood cells (RBCs), fresh frozen plasma (FFP),

[a] Pathology and Laboratory Medicine, University of Pennsylvania Perelman School of Medicine, The Hospital of the University of Pennsylvania, 3400 Spruce Street, Philadelphia, PA 19104, USA; [b] Pathology and Laboratory Medicine, University of Pennsylvania Perelman School of Medicine, The Children's Hospital of Philadelphia, 5136 Main Hospital, 34th and Civic Center Boulevard, Philadelphia, PA 19104-4399, USA
* Corresponding author.
E-mail address: sesok@pennmedicine.upenn.edu

Clin Lab Med 41 (2021) 69–81
https://doi.org/10.1016/j.cll.2020.10.005
0272-2712/21/© 2020 Elsevier Inc. All rights reserved.

cryoprecipitate (CRYO), and platelets. The amount of available blood drives ordering practices and, because most blood banks try to avoid stat delivery requests and charges, these orders are regularly scheduled and transported throughout the day. An example of a minimum RBC inventory and process steps for daily inventory management for a 500-bed tertiary pediatric hospital with a level 1 trauma center, with approximately 20,000 RBC annual transfusions, is given in **Table 1**.

PROCESS STEPS FOR ACTIVE INVENTORY MANAGEMENT

The following are process steps for active inventory management, as adapted from the 2020 standard operating procedures at The Children's Hospital of Philadelphia blood bank laboratory:

- Reconciliation of the available inventory with the available inventory list printed from the laboratory information system (LIS) and resolution of any problems.
- Review of the crossmatched inventory for any units crossmatched on an expired sample and change of the units to available in the LIS with proper change of storage location.
- Reconciliation of the crossmatched and assigned inventory with the crossmatched/assigned inventory list.
- Review of the inventory for expired units and change of status to destroy in the LIS and discard units.
- Visual inspection of the crossmatched inventory for acceptable appearance and documentation of the inspection.
- Review of the available inventory for units that are about to expire and transfer of these units when possible to other regional hospital blood banks.
- Count the RBCs available inventory and notify the blood center of supply needs.
- Count the FFP and platelet inventory to determine the number of units/doses needed to meet the minimum inventory level.
- Visual inspection of the available inventory for acceptability and documentation of the inspection.

In a pediatric blood bank, there may be special requests for ordering and maintaining a supply of fresh universal donor type O-negative RBCs in order to have the units readily available for bleeding patients in need of urgent uncrossmatched blood. These units, less than 7 to less than 10 days old, may be stored in the blood bank or remote refrigerators throughout the hospital where blood may be emergently needed for pediatric patients in the intensive care unit, cardiac intensive care unit, neonatal intensive care unit, and the emergency room. These 1 or 2 units of RBCs are kept for a short duration and, if unused, are rotated back into general inventory and fresh RBCs are replaced in these refrigerators. Fresher blood is preferred to mitigate hyperkalemic reactions in the event a rapid transfusion is needed during an emergency.[1] If fresher

Table 1
Daily inventory red blood cell unit management

Type	O	O−	A	A−	B	B−	AB	AB−	<7 d O-(Weekly)
Leukocyte-reduced red cells	15	8	10	4	4	2	2	2	6

These units are the required minimum daily inventory to support clinical requests. Special requests for directed units, autologous units, and sickle cell antigen–negative units are handled through separate order requests. Fresh cells are ordered based on a weekly schedule.

blood is not available for planned transfusions, most pediatric blood banks wash RBCs, but this cannot be accomplished in the setting of an emergency.[2]

MANUFACTURING ALIQUOTS

Blood transfused to smaller-volume patients is often carefully monitored to avoid fluid overload, and protocols in pediatric blood banks are established to mitigate the risk of transfusion-associated circulatory overload reactions. At doses of 10 to 15 mL/kg for RBCs, 10 to 15 mL/kg for FFP, and 5 to 10 mL/kg for platelets, it is often unavoidable that the requested amount is significantly less than the volume in the unit.[3] For this reason, some pediatric blood banks have pedipacks available from their blood suppliers, which are previously separated product units in smaller storage bags to allow easier unit issuances when an order is placed for a smaller pediatric patient. These pedipacks typically have as much as one-quarter of the volume that would be found in the average unit volume. If these are not available, the blood banks manufacture their own pedipacks by preparing aliquots using a sterile procedure in the blood bank. This option requires a device that heat seals the tubing after the RBCs, FFP, or platelets are transferred to a syringe aliquot or smaller bag. Because it is now considered an open system, these syringes expire at an earlier time than the original parent unit outdate, most often several hours after manufacturing or, at the latest, 24 hours for RBC aliquots and 4 hours for platelet aliquots. The parent unit, if prepared using a sterile procedure and heat sealed, keeps the original unit expiration date. The advantage of this is that the unit may be used over several days to weeks to support a neonate who may require multiple transfusions over time. These designated donor units limit unnecessary exposure of pediatric patients to multiple donors. This practice then helps mitigate infectious disease transmission risks. **Fig. 1** shows an example of a sterile connecting device used to heat seal the original parent unit after an aliquot is prepared in a sterile manner from a single donor platelet unit. Aliquots can be made from any blood product including FFP, RBCs, and platelets.

Although dedicated donor units are good in theory, there may be logistical challenges with assigning units to be transfused to individual pediatric patients over

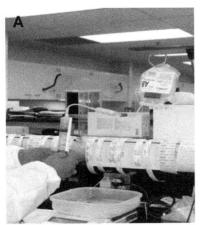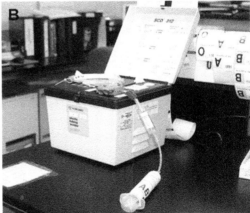

Fig. 1. (*A*) The manufacturing of an aliquot from a platelet product for a pediatric patient requiring less than the amount in the platelet product. (*B*) An example of a sterile docking device that heat seals the container so that the platelet product, or parent product, keeps the original outdate.

time. Assigning units to patients may create workflow issues and potential inventory challenges because blood bank staff must track units available for each patient. For this reason, designated donors are often reserved for the smallest and sickest neonatal patients in whom donor limitation will have the biggest impact. In addition, for older patients who are at risk for multiple donor exposures and developing alloantibodies, when a known transfusion will occur within a few days, requests may be made to split and save half of the RBC unit for future use. This scenario may occur with patients with sickle cell, and reserving the other half of a unit for a later transfusion is a request that may be orderable in the computerized physician order entry system to more readily alert the blood bank of this requirement.

Fresh Blood

A supply of fresh RBCs is necessary for pediatric blood banks to support protocols and patient populations who may be at risk for hyperkalemic reactions. Often these patients are either cardiothoracic patients or craniofacial patients, for whom there is a growing amount of literature that supports the use of fresher blood, in the form of whole blood, for improved hemostasis and reduced donor exposure.[4–7] Although fresh whole blood has historically been used in adult trauma, interest in its potential hemostatic value has expanded into pediatric trauma, where several centers are now exploring its use.[8] Early studies of the safety of uncrossmatched type O cold-stored whole blood are starting to emerge with the use of low titers (<50) anti-A and anti-B in children, with encouraging signs of no increased risk of hemolysis with use among non–group O recipients.[9]

Several important studies have been performed over the years to evaluate the need for fresh RBCs in pediatrics because of concerns of storage lesions causing poorer outcomes following transfusion of older blood. These prospective randomized studies provide insight into the need to balance the clinical concern for fresh blood and inventory management.[10] The ARIPI trial examined the use of fresher versus standard-age inventory blood in premature neonates, and no differences in outcomes in the two groups were noted in terms of morbidity and mortality.[11] Likewise, the RECESS trial examined outcomes in the use of fresher versus older blood in pediatric patients undergoing cardiothoracic surgery and no difference in those two groups was noted.[12] In addition, the ABC-PICU trails examined fresher versus standard older inventory blood in pediatric intensive care patients and did not observe a difference in outcomes in either cohort.[13] These studies indicate that it is unnecessary to keep fresher blood available for all patients and it is unnecessary to avoid transfusion of older blood ($\geq$14 days old). This finding is important for inventory management, because older blood is often selectively used first, because blood is organized on shelves by outdate, in order to avoid excessive wastage by allowing RBCs to expire unused on the shelf.

Storage Lesions of Blood, Additives, Passive Antibodies, and Preventing Adverse Reactions

Although there are different types of anticoagulant/preservative solutions available (AS-1, AS-3, AS-5, Anticoagulant Citrate Phosphate Dextrose Solution (CPD), Citrate-phosphate-dextrose solution with adenine (CPDA)), there is general consensus that washing blood for the removal of these solutions is not necessary, nor is it necessary to limit the inventory in favor of units stored in CPD or CPDA. However, there is a lack of clinical trials to refute or support this practice. Units stored in additive solutions (AS-1, AS-3, AS-5) have lower free potassium levels in the supernatant over time of storage compared with units stored in CPD or CPDA. Because the use of components with additive solutions for transfusion is now widespread in pediatrics, there is no longer a need to keep a separate inventory for patients undergoing more massive transfusion protocols, including extracorporeal membrane oxygenation. However, there is in general a lack of guidelines regarding at-risk populations, including neonates, and large-volume transfusions, which has led to several institution-dependent practices.[14]

The 1 benefit of using a fresher RBC unit is to limit the potassium loads that may be delivered with older or irradiated blood. Irradiation is required to prevent transfusion-associated graft-versus-host disease (TA-GVHD), and, in the best circumstances, RBCs can be irradiated immediately before use to limit the amount of seepage of potassium from RBCs after irradiation.[15] This process is not always logistically possible, and many centers have established protocols for older irradiated units to be washed before transfusion, particularly before transfusion to higher-risk groups requiring massive transfusion, patients with renal failure, or cardiac patients at risk for arrhythmias and hyperkalemic reactions.[16] For this reason, at our institution, RBCs are washed 48 hours after irradiation. However, washed RBCs not used after 24 hours must be discarded, so there is a careful balance with the use of such an approach.

If fresher blood is not available for a patient in whom it is indicated, such as for patients with cardiac disease, renal disease, or massive transfusions, it may be possible to substitute washed RBCs. The indications for washed blood in a pediatric setting are similar to those for adults, including patients with renal failure or multiple repeated allergic reactions, but there are special circumstances that require washing blood in pediatrics.[17,18] One example is washing units to limit the neonate's exposure to passive antibodies. A neonate with a positive direct antiglobulin test caused by passive maternal anti-A, anti-B, or anti-A,B would receive washed type O RBCs by protocol in an attempt to limit the amount of passive antibody from type-specific transfused RBCs, which may further cause RBC destruction. Some institutions extend this practice past the neonatal period to younger, smaller-volume children if incompatible plasma is to be transfused in the setting of a child receiving out-of-group, but compatible, type O RBCs. Washing requires a minimum of 1 hour, so urgent washing is not an option for more time-sensitive transfusions. In this scenario, washing may be waived in the interest of the patient under a medical exception protocol.

As children's age and body size increase, there is less concern about exposure to passive incompatible antibodies. However, investigators have raised this as a continued concern with platelets, and many pediatric hospital transfusion services have adopted approaches to test the antibody titer in donor platelet units and restrict transfusion of out-of-group platelets to only units that have a confirmed low titer of passive antibodies.[19] This restriction is for the purposes of mitigating the risk of a hemolytic reaction caused by passive antibodies. There are a few case reports that have described this situation in a pediatric setting.[20] For pediatric blood banks that are not performing this type of screening, the option of providing saline-replaced, washed, or volume-reduced platelets is another way of limiting incompatible plasma exposure to the recipient to mitigate concerns for a hemolytic reaction.

SPECIAL POPULATIONS FOR INVENTORY MANAGEMENT

In both adult and pediatric blood banking, there are several special populations that require a different approach to inventory management. These populations include patients who have alloantibodies, immunocompromised patients, transplant patients, patients at risk of TA-GVHD, neonates, and patients with sickle cell.

Neonates

One such special population unique to pediatrics is neonates, who cannot themselves produce alloantibodies but may have received passive antibodies from their mothers.

Neonates must receive blood that is not only compatible with their own blood but with their mother's. For example, if a type AB infant is born to a type O mother, that infant may have circulating maternal anti-A,B antibodies. In this situation, the American Association of Blood Banks (AABB) standards require that RBCs lacking the corresponding ABO antigen shall be transfused.[18] Also, if they receive type O blood, then the passive A,B antibodies in the residual donor plasma may cause hemolysis of their own RBCs. In these situations, hospital guidelines may recommend washed type O RBCs. If a neonate's type is unknown and an RBC exchange transfusion is necessary, reconstituted whole blood with type O red cells and type AB plasma may be used. From an inventory management standpoint, these patients are challenging because type O red cells and type AB plasma are in limited supply. Also, for exchange transfusions because of hemolytic disease of the newborn, special antigen-negative units may also be required to avoid the corresponding RBC antigen to the maternal clinically significant antibodies found in the infant's plasma.

Patients with Alloantibodies

In both adult and pediatric blood banking, managing patients with alloantibodies is an important part of inventory and blood bank technologists' resources. Just as in adult patients, patients more than 4 months of age require an active type and screen every 72 hours to determine whether alloantibodies have been produced that require antigen-negative blood. Patients less than 4 months old do not require repeated type and screens because they are not considered capable of forming antibodies, and therefore the only alloantibodies of concern are those obtained from the mother. Depending on the size of the blood bank and its testing capacity, antigen-negative units for specific patients may be purchased from a blood supplier or pulled and tested from the blood bank's own inventory. One study showed that establishing an antigen-negative inventory in a hospital-based blood bank is cost-effective and time efficient, particularly for antigen-negative blood transfused to patients with sickle cell.[21]

Patients with Sickle Cell and β-Thalassemia

These populations require special consideration from an inventory management perspective because they are patients who receive frequent transfusions, are at high risk of forming alloantibodies, and often have a different antigen phenotype from the general donor supply. Specific transfusion considerations for these populations are discussed in more detail in Susan Kuldanek and colleagues' article, "Cellular Therapy in Pediatric Hematologic Malignancies,"elsewhere in this issue, but most centers do some form of antigen matching for these patients. Different strategies include providing RBCs that are stored for 21 days or less; providing units that are E, C, K antigen negative or E, C, K antigen matched; performing extended phenotype matching; and performing molecular matching.[22] Management of these patients requires a close relationship with the patients and their care providers to ensure that the amount of blood required and the timing of administration is well communicated.

Cytomegalovirus Transmission

Cytomegalovirus (CMV) transmission in immunocompromised patients, including transplant patients and premature infants, can have profound clinical consequences, and in blood banking there have been 2 main ways that this risk has been mitigated. The first way is for the donor center to test donors serologically for CMV antibodies and, if they are negative, to mark these units as CMV negative. The second method is to use untested units but to perform prestorage leukoreduction (LR). Because CMV is only present in the white cells, LR of whole blood–derived platelets to fewer than 8.3×10^5 white blood cells (WBCs) per unit and RBCs and single-donor apheresis platelets to fewer than 5×10^6 WBCs per unit is rigorous enough to be considered CMV safe. However, the precise dose of WBCs known to transmit CMV is unknown.[23] These 2 methods are considered to be equivalent in their efficacy by many centers that primarily use LR as their transfusion-transmitted CMV (TT-CMV) mitigation strategy.[24] However, the optimal mitigation strategy to prevent TT-CMV in preterm low-birthweight infants continues to be debated. In some institutions, both LR and CMV serologic testing are performed on all cellular products. A prospective observational comparative effectiveness pilot study was performed using the LR-only strategy and zero cases of TT-CMV were identified. However, the investigators concluded that a larger study and more research in this area are needed.[25]

Leukoreduction

Prestorage LR is performed for multiple reasons, including reducing the risk of CMV transmission, reducing the risk of febrile nonhemolytic transfusion reactions, and reducing the risk of human leukocyte antigen (HLA) alloimmunization. These concerns are of particular importance in immunocompromised patients, in transplant patients, and in patients for whom alloimmunization could prove problematic for their future care, including those who receive frequent platelet transfusions and who are at risk for platelet refractoriness.[26] There is a paucity of studies in pediatric populations on universal LR blood products and there is still variability in practices among hospital transfusion services. A survey on transfusion policies noted that those transfusion services that do not provide universal prestorage LR RBC units to all pediatric patients supply them for (1) neonates only, (2) pediatric hematology oncology patients and neonates, and (3) patients less than 4 months old.[17] However, most (84.8%) survey respondents replied that all RBCs used are leukoreduced before storage.

Irradiation

Irradiation is performed to prevent TA-GVHD, a rare but frequently fatal complication from cellular blood product transfusion, by preventing donor leukocyte DNA replication. Patients at risk of TA-GVHD include patients with very poor CD8 T-cell response, and patients receiving products from an HLA-matched or related donor. Irradiation is indicated for transfusions in patients with hematological transplant and/or congenital immunodeficiency, exchange and intrauterine transfusions, HLA-matched cellular blood product transfusions, and transfusions in preterm infants. Any product containing viable donor lymphocytes, including leukoreduced units, is considered a risk. However, this risk must be weighed in the context of other risks because irradiation has been shown to induce some degradation of RBCs and to increase the potassium level in the product supernatant over time. Strategies for irradiation vary, and include universal irradiation, irradiating only patients assessed to be at high risk for TA-GVHD, irradiating all patients except those deemed to be at high risk for hyperkalemia (such as cardiac surgery patients), and protocols that require either using or washing products that have been irradiated. A recent survey showed that irradiation of cellular blood products continues to be widely disparate across institutions.[27]

Use Management and Product Selection

For inventory management, consideration of the different product types available for transfusion is warranted. For example, there are different platelet products available based on the type of collection, the type of testing for bacteria, and the type of post-collection processing that the platelet may undergo. **Fig. 2** shows an example of an apheresis platelet unit versus a whole blood–derived platelet unit.

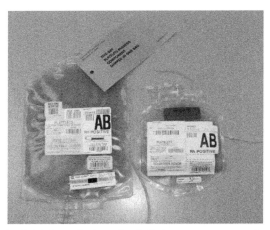

Fig. 2. The apheresis platelet product on the left shows an average size of 200 to 300 mL. The whole blood–derived platelet product on the right shows an average size of 50 to 70 mL.

What is most notable is the size and volume difference between the apheresis and whole blood–derived platelet units. Much like the pedipacks for RBC and FFP, whole blood–derived platelets provide smaller-volume platelet concentrates for smaller-volume patients, avoiding the need to perform additional aliquoting from a larger unit. Both of these types of platelets are cultured at the donor center and both are subject to additional risk mitigation strategies for bacteria as defined by the most recent US Food and Drug Administration (FDA) guidance document.[28] There are widespread practice differences at this time in pediatrics for the best approaches for risk reduction for preventing bacteria transmission from platelets. Some blood banks have adopted the use of point-of-issue bacterial contamination detection testing and plan on increasing the shelf life of platelets to 7 days, as permitted with the use of this method. Other centers have gone to secondary culture, to capture additional bacterial growth missed from the primary culture at the time of collection.[29,30] In addition, other transfusion services have begun to keep an inventory of pathogen-reduced (PR) platelets.[31,32] PR platelets using amotosalen and ultraviolet irradiation (INTERCEPT platelets) are the first FDA-approved pathogen-inactivated platelet product and not only reduce the risk of bacteria transmission but inactivate other viruses as well. Although FDA approved for transfusion, the PIPER postmarketing study is underway with results soon to be analyzed to evaluate acute lung injury in pediatric hematological patients receiving INTERCEPT platelets. Early study reports show no difference in the rate of adverse reactions for patients receiving INTERCEPT platelets compared with conventional platelets.[33] There are some concerns with the transfusion of INTERCEPT platelets in neonates undergoing phototherapy and receiving ultraviolet light therapy, given that INTERCEPT involves use of a synthetic psoralen, which is a photoactive compound. Other concerns are the lower corrected count increment following transfusion of INTERCEPT platelets, which may necessitate transfusion of more units to achieve therapeutic targets.[32] The ramp up to an inventory with 100% PR platelets will take time because of limited national availability. Therefore, hospital transfusion services must be prepared to keep a dual inventory of conventional platelets and PR platelets. In an effort to make conventional platelets safer from the perspective of bacteria transmission, one center implemented PGD testing for all non-PR platelets while in the ramp-up phase.[32] Newer studies are also examining the use of pathogen reduction technology to effectively inactivate WBCs in addition to infectious pathogens so that LR, gamma irradiation, and bacterial screening would not be needed.[34,35]

Patient Blood Management (PBM) largely consists of ensuring that blood is not wasted through expiration, and that products are ordered and used appropriately and in accordance with hospital guidelines. One common strategy hospitals use to guide ordering and transfusion practices is a maximum surgical blood schedule. A maximum surgical blood schedule is a document created through collaboration with surgeons that defines, by specific procedure, the number of units required to meet the needs of most patients who undergo the procedure. The use of a maximum surgical blood schedule helps keep the crossmatch to transfusion ratio low, that is, the ratio of blood ordered to blood transfused. Doing this helps the blood bank correctly anticipate the product needs of scheduled surgeries, and helps surgeons avoid overordering and underusing products. Other benefits include preventing unexpected requests for split and quarter units for a pediatric patient. Although it may seem ideal to provide multiple aliquots for each patient, it may result in wastage if units go unused and are returned to the blood bank.

Many hospitals now have guidelines for blood usage embedded in the electronic ordering system, which allows a blood product order to be flagged for incorrect dosing of products and when certain thresholds are not met. Examples include thresholds for transfusion of RBCs, platelets, and FFP, and, if these are not met and the warning is overridden, the clinician needs to state the reason for the override in a comment section. This system is an example of a prospective audit that attempts to direct clinicians to standard guidelines to avoid unnecessary transfusions. In a recent quality improvement project, clinicians standardized prophylactic platelet transfusion in a pediatric oncology population. They were able to show 85%-90% compliance with orders by using an electronic decision support tool consistent with dosing guidelines established by the PLADO trial.[36,37] Use of a graphic display tool that extracted data from the electronic medical record helped to capture transfusions by service, location, patient service, dose, and platelet trigger value. This method allowed timely feedback to providers on outlier platelet orders. Other institutions have also designed Web-based real-time dashboards to help to improve blood use and decrease RBC unit outdates.[38]

Other examples of auditing are retrospective reviews that are conducted after the blood has already been transfused. Although this is useful for identifying outliers, it does not provide the real-time feedback that may help current inventory management. Because blood components are carefully counted daily and shift to shift, a substantial unnecessary order could cause an influx of inventory that later goes to waste and outdates on the shelf. One way to prevent this is to have a blood bank technologist notify a supervisor or blood bank physician when outlier requests are received in the blood bank. There may even be protocols established to prevent adverse reactions in patients, such as fluid overload, if an order exceeds recommended dosing by weight established in transfusion service policies and procedures. Standard order sets, embedded in the electronic medical record system, may also help to drive best practice and compliance among clinicians.

Blood inventory management is often a balance between shortages and wastage. Hospital transfusion services need to be able to meet clinical demand while minimizing the amount of product expiration. A literature review of models for inventory management in the United Kingdom and the use of case studies at selected hospitals showed that drivers of good inventory performance need not be based on complex inventory models. Instead, basic principles of human resources and training, stock levels and order patterns, transparency of inventories, simple inventory procedures (including a written inventory sheet), a focus on freshness, and internal collaboration within the hospital were all shown to be practical, but simple, approaches to improve wastage.[39]

Managing Remote Inventory for Emergencies and Remote Storage

As pediatric hospitals grow in size and complexity, blood banks may be asked to store blood remotely for ease of issuance and use. This storage may include satellite refrigerators that store uncrossmatched blood for emergency use in emergency rooms and intensive care units or may be a separate remote blood bank located at the same hospital but sufficiently distant from the primary blood bank to warrant a separate location. Inventory management of these remote storage facilities can be managed by the central blood bank with the assistance of the LIS, which allows for tracking and auditing of disposition records of the units. Manual count of units in inventory is still required to reconcile records of RBCs that were crossmatched and made available for issuance versus RBCs that are in inventory and available for distribution. This process requires frequent monitoring of stock in remote refrigerators and units returned to the main storage area, when unused past storage requirements, for example, for freshness criteria. Electronic remote blood issue (ERBI) is also an alternative method for the delivery of RBCs in remote storage and has the advantage of a more controlled way of distributing the units and tracking the person taking the blood.[40] A recent study showed that ERBI at satellite refrigerators improves the efficiency of transfusion by reducing the time for RBCs to reach patients and by reducing time spent by blood bank and clinical staff. This improvement ultimately results in cost savings.[40] In addition to primary specimen barcoding and barcoding of blood products at the time of distribution, the ERBI is an additional safety measure that ensures the right person receives the right blood product. Additional safety devices such as radiofrequency identification (RFID) to track blood products throughout the hospital may provide advantages for inventory management, including the ability to store more information about the blood product, such as temperature, expiration date, and time of collection.[41] RFID also increases transfusion safety, improves inventory management, and decreases product loss, which decreases health care costs through the decrease of product wastage.

In conclusion, inventory management and product selection in pediatric blood banking require a level of complexity beyond that of an adult transfusion service because of the nuances of transfusing neonates and older pediatric patients and the additional risk concerns of hyperkalemia, hypervolemia, alloimmunization, and donor limitation. Best practices require a partnership with the clinical teams to ensure that the procedures are well suited to support proper use of blood components while reducing waste. The essential role of blood bank management and staff is to continuously monitor the supply of blood products to ensure availability to support the clinical demands at the hospital. Fluctuations in day-to-day usage may be anticipated, but long-standing patterns of overinventory and underinventory should be dealt with from the perspective of modifying daily inventory requirements and working closely with the hospital's blood supplier.

ACKNOWLEDGMENTS

The authors thank the blood bank staff and managers and supervisor at The Children's Hospital of Philadelphia for their tireless efforts in the daily management of inventory during the challenging times of the COVID-19 pandemic.

DISCLOSURE

The authors have nothing to disclose.

REFERENCES

1. Lee AC, Redugue LL, Luban NLC, et al. Transfusion-associated hyperkalemic cardiac arrest in pediatric patients receiving massive transfusion. Transfusion 2014;54:244–54.
2. Sesok-Pizzini DA, Pizzini M. Hyperkalemic cardiac arrest in pediatric patients undergoing massive transfusion: unplanned emergencies. Transfusion 2014; 54:4–7.
3. Blood components. In: Wong E, editor. Pediatric transfusion, a physician's handbook. 4th edition. Bethesda (MD): AABB Press; 2015. p. 1–44.
4. Manno CS, Hedberg KW, Kim HC, et al. Comparison of the hemostatic effects of fresh whole blood, stored whole blood, and components after open heart surgery in children. Blood 1991;77(5):930–6.
5. Gruenwald CE, McCrindle BW, Crawford-Lean L, et al. Reconstituted fresh whole blood improves clinical outcomes compared with stored component blood therapy for neonates undergoing cardiopulmonary bypass for cardiac surgery: a randomized controlled trial. J Thorac Cardiovasc Surg 2008;136(6):1442–9.
6. Jobes DR, Sesok-Pizzini D, Friedman D. Reduced transfusion requirement with use of fresh whole blood in pediatric cardiac surgical procedures. Ann Thorac Surg 2015;99(5):1706–11.
7. Thottathil P, Sesok-Pizzini D, Taylor JA, et al. Whole blood in pediatric craniofacial reconstruction surgery. J Craniofac Surg 2017;28(5):1175–8.
8. Yazer MH, Spinella PC. The use of low-titer group O whole blood for the resuscitation of civilian trauma patients in 2018. Transfusion 2018;58:2744–6.
9. Leeper CM, Yazer MH, Cladis FP, et al. Use of uncrossmatched cold-stored whole blood in injured children with hemorrhagic shock. JAMA Pediatr 2018;172(5): 491–2.
10. Dzik W. Fresh blood for everyone: Balancing availability and quality of stored RBCs. Transfus Med 2008;18(4):260–5.
11. Fergusson D, Hutton B, Hogan DL, et al. Effect of fresh red blood cell transfusion on clinical outcomes in premature, very low-birth-weight infants. The ARIP Randomized Trial. JAMA 2012;208(14):1443–51.
12. Steiner ME, Ness PM, Assmann SF, et al. Effects of red-cell storage duration on patients undergoing cardiac surgery. N Engl J Med 2015;372(15):1419–29.
13. Spinella PC, Tucci M, Fergusson DA, et al. Effect of fresh vs standard-issue red blood cell transfusions on multiple organ dysfunction syndrome in crucially ill pediatric patients. A randomized clinical trial. JAMA 2019;322(22):2179–90.
14. Roseff SD, Luban NL, Manno CS. Guidelines for assessing appropriateness of pediatric transfusion. Transfusion 2002;42:1398–413.
15. Weiskopf RB, Schnapp S, Rouine-Rapp K, et al. Extracellular potassium concentrations in red blood cell suspensions after irradiation and washing. Transfusion 2005;45:1295–301.
16. Cardigan R, New HV, Tinegate H, et al. Washed red cells: theory and practice. Vox Sang 07 July 2020 (Online ahead of print). Available at: https://doi-org. proxy.library.upenn.edu/10.1111/vox.12971.
17. Spinella PC, Dressler A, Tucci M, et al. Survey of transfusion policies at US and Canadian children's hospitals in 2008 and 2009. Transfusion 2010;50(11): 2328–35.

18. The AABB Standards Committee. Standards for blood banks and transfusion services. Bethesda (MD): AABB Press; 2020.
19. Josephson Cd, Mullis NC, Van Demark C, et al. Significant numbers of apheresis-derived group O platelet units have "high-titer" anti-A/A,B: implications for transfusion policy. Transfusion 2004;44:805–8.
20. Josephson CD, Castillejo M-I, Grima K, et al. ABO-mismatched platelet transfusions: strategies to mitigate patient exposure to naturally occurring hemolytic antibodies. Transfus Apher Sci 2010;42:83–8.
21. Le N, Harach ME, Kay JK, et al. Establishing an antigen-negative red blood cell inventory in a hospital-based blood bank. Transfusion 2014;54:285–8.
22. Chou St, Alsawas M, Fasano RM, et al. American Society of Hematology 2020 guidelines for sickle cell disease: transfusion support. Blood Adv 2020;4(2):327–55.
23. Weisberg SP, Staley EM, Williams LA, et al. Survey on transfusion-transmitted cytomegalovirus and cytomegalovirus disease mitigation. Arch Pathol Lab Med 2017;141:1705–11.
24. Overview of special products in blood components. In: Wong E, editor. Pediatric transfusion, a physician's handbook. 4th edition. Bethesda (MD): AABB Press; 2015. p. 1–44.
25. Delaney M, Mayock D, Knezevic A, et al. Postnatal cytomegalovirus infection: a pilot comparative effectiveness study of transfusion safety using leukoreduced-only transfusion strategy. Transfusion 2016;56:1945–50.
26. Mendrone A, Fabrone A, Langhi D, et al. Is there justification for universal leukoreduction? Rev Bras Hematol Hemoter 2014;36(4):237.
27. Pritchard AE, Shaz BH. Survey of irradiation practice for the prevention of transfusion-associated graft-versus –host disease. Arch Pathol Lab Med 2016; 140:1092–7.
28. Bacterial risk control strategies for blood collection establishments and transfusion services to enhance the safety and availability of platelets for transfusion. Guidance for Industry. Silver Spring (MD): US Food and Drug Administration; 2019. Available at: https://www.fda.gov/regulatory-information/search-fda-guidance-documents/bacterial-risk-control-strategies-blood-collection-establishments-and-transfusion-services-enhance. Assessed November 9, 2020.
29. Dunbar NM. Modern solutions and future challenges for platelet inventory management. Transfusion 2015;55:2053–6.
30. Harm SK, Szcepiorkowski ZM, Dunbar NM. Routine use of Day 6 or Day 7 platelets with rapid testing: two hospitals assess impact 1 year after implementation. Transfusion 2018;58:938–42.
31. Levy JH, Neal MD, Herman JH. Bacterial contamination of platelets for transfusion: strategies for prevention. Crit Care 2018;22(1):271–8.
32. Rutter S, Snyder EL. How do we...integrate pathogen reduced platelets into our hospital blood bank inventory? Transfusion 2019;59:1628–36.
33. Schulz WL, McPadden J, Gehrie EA. Blood utilization and transfusion reactions in pediatric patients transfused with conventional or pathogen reduced platelets. J Pediatr 2019;209:220–5.
34. Sim J, Tsoi WC, Lee CK, et al. Transfusion of pathogen-reduced platelet components without leukoreduction. Transfusion 2019;59:1953–61.
35. Cid J. Prevention of transfusion-associated graft-versus-host disease with pathogen-reduced platelets with amotosalen and ultraviolet A light: a review. Vox Sang 2017;112(7):607–13.

36. Leibowitz M, Wolfe H, Flynn A, et al. Standardization of prophylactic platelet transfusion dosing in a pediatric oncology population: a quality improvement project. Transfusion 2018;58:2836–40.
37. Slichter SJ, Kaufman RM, Assmann SF, et al. Dose of prophylactic platelet transfusions and prevention of hemorrhage. N Engl J Med 2010;362:600–13.
38. Sharpe C, Quinn J, Watson S, et al. Novel web-based real-time dashboard to optimize recycling and use of red ell units at a large multi-site transfusion service. J Pathol Inform 2014;5:35.
39. Stanger SHW, Yates N, Wilding R, et al. Blood inventory management: hospital best practices. Transfus Med Rev 2012;26(2):153–63.
40. Staples S, Staves J, Davies J, et al. Electronic remote blood issue supports efficient and timely supply of blood and cost reduction: evidence from five hospitals at different stages of implementation. Transfusion 2019;59:1683–91.
41. Coustasse A, Meadows P, Hibner T. Utilizing radiofrequency identification technology to improve safety and management of blood bank supply chains. Telemed J E Health 2015;21(11):938–45.

Evaluation and Management of Coagulopathies and Thrombophilias in Pediatric Patients

HyoJeong Han, MD, Lisa Hensch, MD, Shiu-Ki Rocky Hui, MD,
Jun Teruya, MD, DSc*

KEYWORDS

- Inherited thrombophilia • Acquired thrombophilia • Venous thromboembolism
- Anticoagulation • Congenital coagulopathy • Acquired coagulopathy
- Routine coagulation testing • Developmental hemostasis

KEY POINTS

- Coagulation screening for bleeding and thrombophilia disorders in infants and children provides critical clinical information but can be misleading because of an immature hemostatic system, preanalytical errors, interference, or the presence of acute phase response.
- Hemophilia and von Willebrand disease are congenital coagulopathies that require specialized testing for diagnosis and often require management with factor concentrate or recombinant factor replacement therapy.
- Multiple factor deficiencies can be seen in several acquired coagulopathies, such as disseminated intravascular coagulation, liver disease, vitamin K deficiency, and dilutional coagulopathy. These conditions may require treatment with blood components or prothrombin complex concentrates.
- Initial management of thrombosis is usually initiating therapeutic anticoagulation while laboratory or imaging evaluation is underway.
- Thrombophilia testing is performed in children or adolescents with spontaneous thrombus or unusual site of thrombus.

INTRODUCTION

Evaluation of coagulopathy and thrombophilia among pediatric patients poses significant and unique challenges compared with their adult counterparts. The immature hemostatic system in early childhood and lack of validated pediatric bleeding and thrombotic risk scores highlight part of these difficulties. An accurate personal and

Pathology & Immunology, Baylor College of Medicine, 6621 Fannin Street, Houston, TX
77030, USA
* Corresponding author.
E-mail address: jteruya@bcm.edu

Clin Lab Med 41 (2021) 83–100
https://doi.org/10.1016/j.cll.2020.10.006   labmed.theclinics.com
0272-2712/21/© 2020 Elsevier Inc. All rights reserved.

family hemostasis history can help guide the evaluation process; however, these limitations necessitate an algorithmic approach to the laboratory work-up. This article discusses the evaluation and management of coagulopathies and thrombophilias in pediatric patients.

CONTENT
Acquired or Congenital Coagulopathy

Most screening assays for coagulopathy are performed in citrated, platelet-poor plasma. Although they provide critical information, they are also susceptible to preanalytical errors (ie, clotting, hemolysis, lipemia, and icterus) and interference (ie, lupus anticoagulant, anticoagulants). Screening assays fail to identify all causes of increased bleeding risk, such as defects in platelet function, hyperfibrinolysis, or factor (F) XIII deficiency. Notably, coagulation assays in children are affected by developmental hemostasis, with reference ranges in very young children being significantly different from those in adults.[1] However, the local reference ranges reported at many centers are determined by testing healthy adults rather than children, adding additional challenges.

The identification of bleeding disorders requires a systematic approach, starting with routine coagulation assays including the prothrombin time (PT), activated partial thromboplastin time (aPTT), fibrinogen, and platelet count.[2] These tests should be performed for patients reporting a personal or family history of bleeding, or those suspected to have developed an acquired coagulopathy in the setting of sepsis, liver disease, trauma, or prolonged illness (**Fig. 1**, **Table 1**).

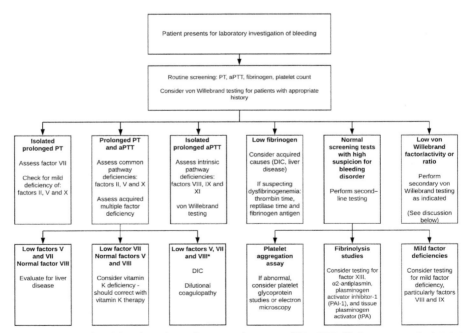

Fig. 1. Testing algorithm based on the screening tests (PT, aPTT, fibrinogen, and platelet count). DIC, disseminated intravascular coagulation. *Note: Factor VIII can be normal or increased in these settings secondary to the acute phase response.

Table 1
Causes of bleeding associated with prolonged prothrombin time and activated partial thromboplastin time

Isolated Prolonged PT	Isolated Prolonged aPTT	Prolonged PT and aPTT	Causes of Bleeding Without PT/aPTT Prolongation
FVII deficiency	Hemophilia A (FVIII deficiency)	Disseminated intravascular coagulation	FXIII deficiency
Mild common pathway factor deficiency (II, V, and X), fibrinogen deficiency	Hemophilia B (FIX deficiency)	Dilutional coagulopathy	von Willebrand disease
Early vitamin K deficiency	Hemophilia C (FXI deficiency)	Liver synthetic dysfunction	Platelet dysfunction
Early liver synthetic dysfunction	von Willebrand disease	Marked vitamin K deficiency	Mild deficiency of FVIII, FIX, and FXI
Direct Xa inhibitor	Acquired FVIII, FIX, or FXI inhibitors	Common pathway factor deficiency (FII, FV, and FX), severe fibrinogen deficiency	α2-antiplasmin deficiency and other causes of hyperfibrinolysis
—	Heparin	Warfarin or direct thrombin inhibitor, DOAC (not always)	Collagen vascular diseases (ie, Ehlers-Danlos syndrome)
—	—	Increased tissue factor pathway inhibitor, FV Amsterdam or East Texas bleeding disorder	DOAC

Abbreviation: DOAC, direct oral anticoagulant.

Congenital Coagulopathies

Hemophilia A

Hemophilia A is an X-linked disorder that results in varying degrees of FVIII deficiency. Its frequency is estimated to be around 1 in 5000 male births. The clinical manifestations of hemophilia A can range from mild to life threatening.[3] Although female carriers were historically thought to be clinically asymptomatic, recent studies have shown that female carriers can have significant bleeding symptoms, including heavy menstrual bleeding and postpartum hemorrhage.[4] The diagnosis of hemophilia A is based on the level of FVIII activity: severe, less than 1%; moderate, 1% to 5%; and mild, 6% to 40%.

Historically, hemophilia diagnosis is based on the 1-stage factor activity assay, but there are patients with discrepant FVIII activity between the 1-stage versus the 2-stage factor assays.[5] These patients with discrepant hemophilia have more severe bleeding symptoms than the 1-stage activity level may otherwise suggest.[6] von Willebrand disease (VWD) should also be considered in the differential and must be ruled out when diagnosing hemophilia A. Management of hemophilia is focused on replacement therapy using recombinant FVIII. Blood products are no longer used routinely in hemophilia A treatment, with the rare exception of cryoprecipitate when factor concentrates are not available. The therapy targets depend on the procedures involved and range from 50% for dental procedures to more than 80% for major surgeries.[7] Recently, clotting factor mutations resistant to clot inhibitors (emicizumab) have been used, and anti-thrombin small interfering RNA and anti–tissue factor pathway inhibitor are being studied.

Hemophilia B

Hemophilia B is an X-linked disorder with deficiency in FIX. Its incidence is approximately 1 in 25,000 male births. As in hemophilia A, the severity of the disease ranges from mild to life threatening based on FIX activity level. The diagnosis of hemophilia B is based on the level of FIX activity: severe, less than 1%; moderate, 1% to 5%; and mild, 6% to 40%. To further complicate the diagnosis, FIX activity does not reach adult levels during infancy and early childhood. In addition, FIX is a vitamin K–dependent factor, so careful consideration of these factors is required before making a diagnosis of hemophilia B, especially in early childhood.[8] Management is based on replacement therapy using recombinant FIX. However, unlike FVIII, there are no appropriate blood component alternatives for FIX replacement. Targets depend on the clinical situations with dental procedures at 50% and major surgeries at less than 80%.[7]

Hemophilia C

FXI deficiency is inherited in an autosomal recessive pattern and is reported in approximately 1:1 million patients. Most bleeding in FXI deficiency is injury related, and bleeding is more severe at sites with high amounts of fibrinolysis (urinary tract, mouth, and nose).[9] Unlike the bleeding seen in hemophilia A and hemophilia B, the phenotype of bleeding in FXI deficiency does not correlate with FXI activity levels.[10] Treatment options for FXI deficiency generally include fresh frozen plasma (FFP) and tranexamic acid. FXI concentrates are not available in the United States, but are available in certain European countries. For surgical procedures, transfusion of FFP should be given to target a level of 40%, being mindful of the potential for volume overload. Tranexamic acid can be used for minor dental procedures and menorrhagia.[9]

von Willebrand disease

VWD is the most common heritable bleeding disorder across all ethnic groups and genders, affecting up to 1% of population. The bleeding symptoms and severity vary depending on the level and type of deficiency and the gender of the patient.[11] Because of this wide range of clinical symptoms, the diagnosis of VWD depends greatly on the laboratory findings.[12] **Table 2** shows individual tests that may be included in a von Willebrand panel.

An additional complexity to the VWD work-up is the fact that von Willebrand factor (VWF) is an acute phase reactant, therefore a normal VWF level cannot definitively rule out the diagnosis. Repeat testing is often necessary.

VWD can be broadly divided into quantitative (type 1 and type 3) and qualitative disorders (type 2). Quantitative diseases are disorders where the defects are in the amount of VWF present. Type 1 disease has a level less than 30%, whereas type 3 disease has a level less than 3%. Despite the decreased level of VWF antigen, the function of VWF remains intact in type 1 and type 3 disorders. In contrast, the type 2 VWDs all share the commonality of having functional defects, including defects in coagulation or FVIII carrier function. The general diagnostic criteria for the common subtypes of VWD are listed in **Table 3**.[13]

As in hemophilia, the management for VWD is replacement. Historically, cryoprecipitate has been the replacement therapy of choice. However, VWF concentrates have been gaining popularity in recent years. VWF concentrates have the advantage of less infectious risk, standardized dosing, and less thrombotic potential. For minor procedures, with the exception of type 2B VWD, desmopressin (DDAVP) may be used to

Table 2
von Willebrand panel

Assay	Clinical Utility
VWF antigen	ELISA or latex immunoassay method for quantitative measurement of VWF
VWF activity	Measures VWF ability to interact with platelet GPIb receptors. Ristocetin cofactor assay is often referred to as the historical standard for VWF activity evaluation. However, ristocetin-independent methodologies are now rapidly gaining and have advantages compared with ristocetin-dependent assay
VWF activity to VWF antigen ratio	Calculation used to determine whether discrepancy exists between the activity and antigen level. A low ratio (<0.7) indicates coagulation function defect in VWF ability to interact with GPIb receptor[13]
VWF multimer	Electrophoresis-based method evaluating VWF multimer distribution
VWF collagen binding	ELISA-based method evaluating the ability of VWF to bind to collagen. However, the clinical use is not to determine collagen binding ability of VWF but to evaluate the presence or absence of high-molecular-weight multimers
FVIII	A PTT-based activity assay to determine the FVIII activity. The utility in a VWF work-up is to determine the ability of VWF to function as an FVIII carrier protein. An increase in FVIII suggests testing during acute phase reaction

Abbreviations: ELISA, enzyme-linked immunosorbent assay; GPIb, glycoprotein Ib; VWF, von Willebrand factor.

temporarily increase the baseline VWF level. However, if the target must be maintained beyond a few hours, replacement therapy is required because repeat DDAVP dosing produces tachyphylaxis. The targets for replacement range from 60% for dental procedures to more than 80% for major surgeries.[14]

Acquired Coagulopathies

Disseminated intravascular coagulation

Disseminated intravascular coagulation (DIC) is characterized by systemic activation of the coagulation system leading to both bleeding and clotting complications as well as organ failure. DIC is a clinicopathologic diagnosis requiring both clinical and

Table 3
Classification of von Willebrand disease

Subtype	FVIII	VWF Antigen	VWF Activity	Activity/ Antigen Ratio	Multimer
Type 1	Low to normal	<30%	<30%	>0.7	Normal
Type 2A	Low to normal	Low to normal	Low	<0.7	Missing large multimer
Type 2B	Low to normal	Low to normal	Low	<0.7	Missing large multimer
Type 2M	Low to normal	Low to normal	Low	<0.7	Normal
Type 2N	Significantly lower than VWF Antigen	Low to normal	Low to normal	>0.7	Normal
Type 3	<10%	<3%	<3%	Not applicable	Absent

laboratory criteria. Predisposing conditions for DIC include sepsis/infection, malignancy, traumatic brain injury, incompatible blood transfusion, trauma, large vascular abnormalities, drowning, and various toxic exposures.[15] The PT, aPTT, platelet count, and fibrinogen levels provide critical information about the extent of coagulation activation and consumption, and the D-dimer provides information about the extent of fibrin formation and lysis.[15] Traditionally, DIC presents with prolonged PT/aPTT, low platelet count, and low fibrinogen level. However, these changes may not be uniformly present in the initial stages in DIC. In particular, fibrinogen level may increase as part of the acute phase reaction before decreasing precipitously. The platelet count may remain in the normal range while showing a downward trend. The aPTT may be paradoxically shortened because of increased FVIII at the onset of DIC, although FVIII levels should become normal or decreased as consumption continues.

The International Society of Thrombosis and Hemostasis (ISTH) has developed a scoring system for DIC based on presence of underlying conditions, fibrin markers, PT, platelet count, and fibrinogen level.[15] However, evaluation of the sensitivity and specificity for DIC in pediatric patients is lacking. A study performed by Soundar and colleagues[16] reported a sensitivity and specificity of 0.65 and 0.43, respectively, when the ISTH scoring system was compared with autopsy findings of DIC in pediatric patients. In the same study, modification of these criteria, including serial platelet and fibrinogen measurements, increased sensitivity to 0.82, although specificity was significantly lower than that of the ISTH system. The study also highlighted the importance of serial measurements to identify evolving DIC.[16]

Management of DIC should focus on the following:[15,17]

1. Treat the underlying condition
2. Perform serial monitoring
3. Transfuse platelets for counts less than 50,000/μL if bleeding or planned invasive procedure
4. Consider plasma transfusion for bleeding patients with PT/aPTT greater than 1.5 times normal range
5. Transfusion support with cryoprecipitate for fibrinogen level less than 150 mg/dL in bleeding patients
6. Consider anticoagulation with heparin when thrombosis predominates or purpura fulminans is present
7. In some countries, antithrombin concentrate, recombinant thrombomodulin, or gabexate mesilate (a synthetic serine proteinase inhibitor) may be used

Vitamin K deficiency

Vitamin K, a fat-soluble vitamin, is required for γ-carboxylation of FII, FVII, FIX, and FX. In the absence of vitamin K, these factors circulate in inactive forms. Inactive vitamin K–deficient factors are known as protein induced by vitamin K absence. Vitamin K deficiency (VKD) can be congenital or associated with a variety of clinical settings, including malabsorption, poor dietary intake, prolonged vomiting or diarrhea, prolonged antibiotic therapy, and cholestasis. Newborns are particularly susceptible to low vitamin K because of poor placental transfer and low vitamin K content in breast milk.[18] VKD in neonates is classified into 3 time periods:

1. Early (<24 hours), caused by maternal factors or congenital deficiency and characterized by cephalohematoma, intracranial bleeding, or umbilical bleeding
2. Classic (2–7 days), caused by delayed feeding or poor breast milk content characterized by gastrointestinal, umbilical, ear/nose/throat bleeding or bleeding from venipuncture

3. Late (2–6 months), caused by low breast milk content, low vitamin K intake, and/or hepatobiliary disease and mostly characterized by intracranial bleeding[18]

However, VKD can occur at any age, and clinicians should be suspicious for the development of VKD in any patient with prolonged hospitalization. The early stages of VKD may have a prolonged PT only because of the shorter half-life of FVII and increased sensitivity of some PT reagents to common pathway factor deficiencies. However, as VKD persists, both the PT and aPTT become prolonged.

Management of VKD depends on the clinical presentation. Vitamin K can be given orally, subcutaneously, intramuscularly, or intravenously. All routes of administration lead to a reduction in PT/INR over 24 hours. Intravenous administration of vitamin K has been associated with anaphylaxis, but works the most rapidly. For patients who are not bleeding and are not in need of an urgent invasive procedure, oral administration of vitamin K is acceptable. Subcutaneous and intramuscular injections of vitamin K should be avoided when the PT is significantly prolonged, because this may lead to unwanted bleeding at the injection site. Previously, FFP was used for correction of VKD. However, the volume of FFP required to correct this deficiency can be significant and increases the risk for volume overload. Prothrombin complex concentrate (PCC) can also be used for urgent reversal of VKD in the setting of active hemorrhage or urgent need for procedure. Note that, unless given with vitamin K, the effects of PCCs are temporary.

Liver failure
Acute or chronic liver disease is a common cause for acquired coagulopathy in pediatric patients. Liver dysfunction or failure can arise from a variety of settings, including infections, metabolic diseases, shock, autoimmune disease, various drugs, malignancies, and even thrombosis.[19] Hemostatic changes seen in liver disease are driven by the following 5 factors:

1. Decreased synthesis of coagulation proteins and thrombopoietin
2. Systemic intravascular coagulation leading to consumption
3. Endothelial cell activation
4. Hyperfibrinolysis
5. Increased platelet pooling in the spleen[20]

Management in this setting is confounded by the concept of the so-called balanced coagulopathy seen in liver disease. That is, although levels of many synthetic clotting factors are decreased, anticoagulant proteins are also decreased in this setting. The fibrinolytic cascade is also altered. **Table 4** outlines these changes. Platelet counts are often decreased in the setting of liver disease because of decreased thrombopoietin and splenomegaly. Screening tests (PT, aPTT, and fibrinogen) fail to show the balance seen in liver disease. Therefore, coagulation in this setting may be better assessed by global hemostasis assays such as rotational thromboelastometry (ROTEM) or thromboelastography (TEG).[19] Care should be taken to avoid overcorrection in patients without clinical evidence of bleeding. Children, particularly neonates and infants, are susceptible to volume overload. Transfusion of large amounts of FFP can lead to increased venous pressure in patients with liver disease and may lead to bleeding.[20]

Nonetheless, acute circumstances such as bacterial infection, ruptured esophageal varices, and/or concurrent renal failure can tip the balance toward bleeding. Transfusion support in patients with bleeding liver usually involves FFP, cryoprecipitate, and platelets. If the volume can be tolerated, FFP is an appropriate choice as a source of all coagulation proteins. PCCs can be considered for off-label use in this setting,

Table 4 Coagulation changes in liver disease		
Changes in Procoagulant Proteins	**Changes in Anticoagulant Proteins**	**Changes in Antifibrinolytic Proteins**
Decreased fibrinogen and factors FII, FV, FVII, FIX, FX, and FXI	Decreased protein C	Decreased α2-antiplasmin and thrombin-activatable fibrinolysis inhibitor[21,22]
Increased FVIII	Decreased protein S	FXIII decreased in some patients[23]
Increased VWF, decreased ADAMTS-13	Decreased antithrombin	Increased tissue plasminogen activator

Abbreviation: ADAMTS-13, a disintegrin and metalloproteinase with a thrombospondin type 1 motif, member 13.

particularly for patients with concerns for volume overload, and has been shown to be effective in correcting coagulopathy associated with liver disease.[24,25] However, PCCs may be more thrombogenic than FFP, and larger clinical trials in the pediatric population are needed to establish safety and dosing in this setting. Replacement should be guided by ROTEM or TEG in addition to routine coagulation assays, and complete correction of PT/INR may not be required to achieve adequate hemostasis as determined by viscoelastic testing. Fibrinogen should be maintained at least greater than 100 mg/dL; the authors use a target of 150 to 200 mg/dL in actively bleeding patients depending on the extent of hemorrhage. Note that cryoprecipitate also supplies concentrated amounts of FVIII and VWF, which are already increased in liver disease, and in some settings (preexisting thrombosis) fibrinogen concentrate may be a favorable alternative. As with PCCs, this use is off label, and further studies are warranted. Platelet counts should be maintained at greater than 50,000/µL in the setting of active bleeding. In the absence of contraindications such as thrombosis or urinary tract bleeding, tranexamic acid should be considered for patients with known or suspected hyperfibrinolysis, although studies are ongoing to better evaluate safety and efficacy in the setting of liver disease.[26]

Trauma and dilutional coagulopathy

Injury is the leading cause of mortality in children. Coagulopathy in trauma is multifactorial. A retrospective study performed by Hendrickson and colleagues[27] (2012) showed that abnormalities in platelet count, PT, and aPTT in pediatric patients with trauma correlated with mortality. In addition, if they survived, patients with coagulopathy on arrival required longer intensive care unit admission and had more ventilator days. Pediatric patients with trauma should be assessed on arrival for presence of coagulopathy using PT, aPTT, fibrinogen, platelet count, and D-dimer. Coagulation abnormalities should be corrected using laboratory-directed transfusion therapy whenever possible. For patients presenting with massive hemorrhage, initial resuscitation should begin with a 1:1 to 1:2 ratio of FFP to red blood cells (RBCs) to prevent dilutional coagulopathy. Patients who had initial resuscitation with large amounts of crystalloid solutions may require additional FFP up front to catch up to their coagulopathy. Coagulopathy can also be compounded by acidosis and hypocalcemia. Efforts should be made to monitor and correct acidosis, which can lead to hyperkalemia. Ionized calcium levels must also be maintained in the setting of massive hemorrhage. ROTEM or TEG should be considered in these settings for rapid assessment of coagulation status when standard assays are not rapidly available to aid in the transition to goal-directed therapy. Hyperfibrinolysis can occur in the setting of trauma.

Tranexamic acid was shown in the PED-TRAX (pediatric trauma and tranexamic acid) study to reduce mortality in pediatric trauma[28] and should be considered for use within 3 hours of injury.

Acquired von Willebrand syndrome

Acquired von Willebrand syndrome (AVWS) is a collection of acquired VWF quantitative or qualitative defects secondary to underlying diseases. Dozens of diseases have been documented to be associated with AVWS, including cardiovascular abnormalities and malignancies with mechanisms ranging from shear force destruction to autoantibodies.[29] The laboratory findings often mimic type 2A VWD where large molecular multimers are absent. However, type 1 VWD such as AVWS has also been reported.[30] Although AVWS shares some of the same laboratory findings as congenital VWDs, the clinical symptoms vary from asymptomatic to serious. In addition, the degree of VWF abnormalities in AVWS and clinical severity do not directly correlate. These aspects create unique challenges in treating patients with AVWS. The general recommendation is to treat only if the patient is symptomatic via VWF replacement or with DDAVP.[31]

Factor inhibitors

Factor-specific inhibitors are occasionally found among patients with congenital factor deficiency who subsequently developed inhibitors from chronic factor replacement therapy. These inhibitors are alloantibodies formed by patients who do not natively produce these coagulation proteins.[32] However, acquired factor deficiency can also develop if an autoantibody against a specific coagulation factor is present. The most commonly reported acquired factor deficiency is acquired hemophilia A, in which the patient develops an autoantibody against FVIII. Acquired hemophilia A has been associated with malignancies, infections, and autoimmune diseases.[33] Autoimmune diseases such as systemic lupus erythematosus have also been associated with FXIII[34,35] and FII[36,37] deficiencies. The latter condition is also known as lupus anticoagulant hypoprothrombinemia syndrome.[36,37] The diagnosis of acquired factor deficiency requires foremost the recognition of such disorders by clinicians. The combination of clinical bleeding symptoms, which are often sudden onset and severe, along with the unexpected prolongation of PT and/or aPTT should prompt further work-up to identify the factor responsible. Treatment of acquired factor deficiencies requires immunosuppression. However, in some rare and severe cases, patients may require bypassing agents when simple factor replacement and blood components therapies are ineffective.

EVALUATION AND MANAGEMENT OF PEDIATRIC THROMBOSIS

Thrombosis is not common in children, but the incidence has been increasing. The Pediatric Health Information System database noted a 70% increase in pediatric venous thromboembolism (VTE) in the United States from 2001 to 2007, with a higher incidence in hospitalized children.[38] The increase in incidence is caused by the improved attention to and recognition of VTE symptoms; advancement of medicine has resulted in improved survival of children with chronic conditions and increased use of central venous catheters (CVCs).[38,39] Thrombosis typically occurs because of the underlying condition, such as CVC, sepsis, and dehydration.[39] Children can also present with a spontaneous clot prompting thrombophilia evaluation. Different types of thrombophilia, evaluation, and initial management in pediatric patients are discussed next.

Clinical Presentation

Pediatric patients are usually diagnosed with thrombus because the clot is symptomatic or incidentally identified during evaluation for another problem (eg, routine echocardiogram showing incidental thrombus in one of the heart chambers). Signs and symptoms of clot depend on the location of the thrombus, and the diagnosis is confirmed with imaging (**Table 5**).[39]

Risk Factors for Thrombosis

In neonates and children, thrombosis usually develops because of underlying disease or because of a provoked event (eg, CVC placement, catheterization). The most common cause of provoked thrombosis is the CVC.[38] Other risk factors for thrombosis include sepsis, mechanical ventilation, congenital heart disease, and dehydration.[39] Neonates and children can also develop spontaneous thrombus because of inherited thrombophilia or other causes, which are discussed next.

Thrombophilia Conditions and Laboratory Work-up

When a child develops thrombus because of a provoking event such as the presence of CVC, evaluation of thrombophilia is not suggested. Prior studies have shown that thrombophilia is found less frequently in neonates and children with catheter-associated thrombosis.[40] However, when a child develops spontaneous thrombus that cannot be explained by the clinical risk factors, thrombophilia evaluation is warranted.[38,39] **Table 6** lists thrombophilia disorders and their evaluation.[38,41]

Initial thrombophilia evaluation includes inherited thrombophilias, as listed in **Table 6**. Additional testing is considered in the following situations.

Antiphospholipid antibody syndrome

Children with antiphospholipid antibody syndrome (APS) commonly present with lower extremity deep vein thrombosis (DVT), pulmonary embolism (PE), or both.[42] APS should also be considered in:

Table 5 Signs and symptoms of thrombosis		
Location of Clot	**Presenting Symptoms**	**Radiographic Diagnosis**
Venous thrombus in limbs	Swelling, pain, and/or redness	Venous ultrasonography with Doppler
Arterial thrombus in limbs	Cool limbs, diminished or absent pulse	Arterial ultrasonography with Doppler
Cerebral venous sinus thrombosis	Headache, nausea and/or vomiting, lethargy, change in mental status	CT venography or MR venography of head/brain
Pulmonary embolism	Chest pain, shortness of breath, pleuritis	CT angiography, VQ scan
Thrombus in the heart	Chest pain, shortness of breath, pleuritis	Echocardiogram
Portal vein thrombosis	Abdominal pain, nausea and/or vomiting, anorexia	Right upper quadrant ultrasonography with Doppler
Renal vein thrombosis	Hematuria, abdominal mass, abdominal pain, thrombocytopenia	Renal ultrasonography with Doppler or CT abdomen/pelvis with IV contrast

Abbreviations: CT, computed tomography; IV, intravenous; MR, magnetic resonance; US, ultrasonography; VQ, ventilation-perfusion.

Table 6
Types of thrombophilia and evaluation

Thrombotic Types	Thrombophilia Trait	Evaluation
Inherited Thrombophilia	• Factor V Leiden	• Polymerase chain reaction
	• Prothrombin G20210A mutation	• Polymerase chain reaction
	• Antithrombin deficiency	• Chromogenic or clotting assay
	• Protein C deficiency	• Chromogenic or clotting assay
	• Protein S deficiency	• Clotting assay, immunoturbidimetric assay (free protein S)
	• Hyperhomocysteinemia	• Enzyme immunoassay
	• Elevated lipoprotein (a)	• Immunoassay
Acquired Thrombophilia	• Antiphospholipid antibody syndrome /catastrophic antiphospholipid syndrome	• PTT, DRVVT, hexagonal phase phospholipid neutralization test, ELISA assay for IgG and IgM antibodies directed against cardiolipin and β2 glycoprotein I
	• Heparin-Induced Thrombocytopenia	• Enzyme immunoassay +/- serotonin release assay
	• Paroxysmal nocturnal hemoglobinuria	• Flow cytometry (CD55 and CD59)
Anatomic predisposition	• May-Thurner Anomaly	• CT or MR venography or catheter-based venography
	• Paget-Schroetter syndrome	• CT or MR venography

Abbreviations: CD, cluster of differentiation; DRVVT, dilute Russell's viper venom time; Ig, immunoglobulin.

- Preadolescent children with thrombus[42,43]
- Thrombosis in an unusual site, such as stroke, transient ischemic attack, adrenal infarct[42,43]
- Recurrent thrombosis with prolonged aPTT[42]

Diagnosis of APS is made when the patient has thrombosis with positive antiphospholipid antibodies (positive lupus anticoagulant and/or anticardiolipin antibodies [immunoglobulin (Ig) G or IgM] and/or anti–β2-glycoprotein I antibodies [IgG or IgM]) on 2 or more consecutive occasions separated by a minimum of 12 weeks.[38] Of note, lupus anticoagulant (LA) may be falsely positive when C reactive protein level is increased and falsely positive or negative during anticoagulation treatment.[41] However, anticardiolipin and anti–β2-glycoprotein antibody results are not affected by anticoagulation.[41] Therefore, results should be interpreted carefully.

Catastrophic antiphospholipid antibody syndrome

Catastrophic antiphospholipid antibody syndrome (CAPS) is a rare but severe form of APS where the patient presents with multiple organ thromboses developing within 7 days with persistently positive antiphospholipid antibodies.[42] These patients are critically ill with multiorgan failure (ie, acute renal failure, diffuse alveolar hemorrhage, encephalopathy) requiring intensive care.[42]

May-Thurner anomaly

The left common iliac vein is chronically compressed between an overlying right common iliac artery and an underlying vertebral body, resulting in venous congestion, stasis, and thrombosis.[38] Patients present with left lower extremity swelling, pain, and claudication.[38] Ultrasonography (US) with Doppler reveals extensive thrombus in the left leg and computed tomography (CT) or magnetic resonance (MR) venography usually reveals left common iliac vein compression.

Paget-Schroetter syndrome (venous thoracic outlet syndrome)

Repetitive motion of the upper extremity leads to recurrent injury, endothelial damage, and extrinsic compression of the subclavian vein causing VTE.[38] This syndrome is often seen in baseball pitchers where repetitive throwing leads to compression and thrombosis of the subclavian vein. Patients present with upper extremity pain and/ or swelling. Ultrasonography with Doppler reveals subclavian vein thrombus, and CT or MR venography usually reveals stenosis or compression of subclavian vein at the costoclavicular junction.

Paroxysmal nocturnal hemoglobinuria

This disorder is caused by a somatic mutation in the phosphatidylinositol glycan A gene in hematopoietic stem cells leading to reduction or absence of glycosylphosphatidylinositol (GPI) anchor protein on the surface of blood cells.[44,45] Absence of GPI anchor proteins on blood cells causes uncontrolled complement activation leading to thrombosis and RBC lysis.[45] Therefore, patients present with thrombosis, intravascular hemolysis (increased lactate dehydrogenase level, reticulocytosis, undetectable haptoglobin, hemoglobinuria) and anemia or pancytopenia.[44,45] Diagnosis of paroxysmal nocturnal hemoglobinuria (PNH) is made by high-sensitivity flow cytometry, which reveals loss of cluster of differentiation (CD) 55 and CD59 expression on erythrocytes and loss of GPI-linked structures on neutrophils and monocytes.[45]

Heparin-induced thrombocytopenia

Heparin-induced thrombocytopenia (HIT) typically presents with platelet count decrease of greater than or equal to 50% of the patient's baseline about 5 to 10 days after heparin initiation and is associated with thrombosis (arterial and/or venous).[44] Using the 4T score can help clinicians recognize possible HIT and allow providers to stop all heparin products and initiate laboratory testing.[44,46] Laboratory testing includes antibody-based enzyme immunoassay (very sensitive test that can rule out HIT if the test is negative) and the serotonin release assay (a functional assay that confirms HIT).[44]

Thrombophilia test results in neonates may be abnormal because neonatal factor levels are different from those of older children.[39,41] Infants less than 6 months of age have balanced coagulation and anticoagulation, but the concentration of many factors are variable during development.[39,41] More specifically, levels of the following factors are low, and even lower in premature neonates[39,41]:

- Procoagulants: FII, FVII, FIX, and FX
- Anticoagulants: protein S, protein C, and antithrombin

Thrombophilia testing during acute illness may show abnormal results.[41] This finding can occur when the evaluation is obtained during:

- Acute thrombosis: antithrombin, protein C, and protein S levels may be low; antiphospholipid antibody levels may be increased[41]
- Acute inflammation: FVIII and lipoprotein (a) levels may be increased[41]

- Vitamin K antagonist therapy: protein C and protein S levels are low[41]

Therefore, repeat testing when the child is well is recommended.[41] In contrast, molecular mutation testing (FV Leiden and prothrombin G20210A mutation) is not affected, even during acute illness, and can be obtained at any time.[41]

Management

Initial management of acute thrombosis usually begins with initiation of therapeutic anticoagulation to slow or stop thrombus progression and embolization.[38] Some exceptions are neonates or children with protein C, protein S, or antithrombin deficiencies who present with purpura fulminans, extensive large vessel thrombosis, or DIC.[41] These patients require replacement with plasma-derived concentrate (protein C or antithrombin) or plasma in addition to anticoagulation.[41] The following anticoagulants are available in pediatric patients: unfractionated heparin (UFH), low-molecular-weight heparin (LMWH), fondaparinux, bivalirudin, argatroban, vitamin K antagonist (VKA), and direct oral anticoagulant (DOAC). In general, the American Society of Hematology (ASH) guidelines recommend therapeutic anticoagulation in patients with symptomatic DVT or PE, and suggests either starting or not starting anticoagulation in patients with asymptomatic DVT or PE (treatment should be individualized).[47] The choice of anticoagulant depends on bleeding risk and comorbidities.[47] Usually children are started on UFH or LMWH. UFH is preferred in patients going for surgery and those with an increased risk of bleeding because of its short half-life and reversal with protamine.[39,47,48] UFH and LMWH are monitored using the following:

- UFH: goal anti-Xa activity of 0.35 to 0.7 units/mL or an aPTT range that correlates to the therapeutic anti-Xa range[39,48]
- LMWH: goal anti-Xa activity of 0.5 to 1.0 units/mL[39,48]

Initial management may vary depending on the thrombophilia disorder, which is discussed later. Duration of anticoagulation is not discussed here because the length of therapy may vary depending on the patient's clinical status. General guidelines on duration of treatment can be found in ASH[47] and CHEST guidelines.[48] In neonates, providers may choose to treat or observe the thrombus depending on the following comorbidities: age (prematurity increases risk of intraventricular hemorrhage); bleeding risk; severity of thrombus; and underlying condition, such as sepsis or congenital heart disease.[39] Before initiating anticoagulation, head ultrasonography should be performed if a recent head ultrasonography result is not available. Usually neonates are started on UFH because of its short half-life and available reversal agent.[39] However, UFH bolus may not be advisable in neonates with significant bleeding risk such as prematurity.[39] LMWH is an option if the bleeding risk is not increased.[39] UFH or LMWH dosing should be monitored and adjusted closely to achieve therapeutic goal (as mentioned earlier).[39,48] Thrombectomy or catheter-directed thrombolysis is considered only if the thrombus is life, limb, or organ threatening.[39] It is done by interventional radiology (IR), vascular surgery, or plastic surgery.

May-Thurner anomaly
Initiate therapeutic anticoagulation with either UFH or LMWH and consult IR.[38] IR will perform thrombectomy and/or catheter-directed thrombolysis followed by stent placement to prevent left iliac vein compression.[38]

Paget-Schroetter syndrome

Initiate therapeutic anticoagulation with either UFH or LMWH and consult IR and surgery.[38] IR will perform thrombectomy and/or catheter-directed thrombolysis. Once the patient is stable and on therapeutic anticoagulation, surgery will resect the first rib on the involved side to prevent compression of the vein.[38]

Antiphospholipid antibody syndrome

Initiate therapeutic anticoagulation with either UFH or LMWH followed by long-term anticoagulation with VKA such as warfarin.[42] Note, aPTT cannot be used to monitor UFH therapy if aPTT is prolonged because of the presence of LA. Although it is less common than aPTT, if baseline PT is also prolonged because of LA, INR cannot be used to monitor warfarin effect. Of note, if IgG or IgM antiprothrombin antibody is present, PT is also prolonged because of a decreased FII level (ie, lupus anticoagulant hypoprothrombinemia syndrome). Data on use of DOACs in patients with APS are limited.[44] DOAC is not recommended in triple-positive cases (positive lupus anticoagulant, anticardiolipin, and anti–β2-glycoprotein antibodies) because a prior clinical trial showed more thrombotic events with a DOAC group compared with a warfarin group.[44]

Catastrophic antiphospholipid antibody syndrome

In addition to initiating therapeutic anticoagulation with UFH, patients are started on corticosteroid and therapeutic plasma exchange (TPE) because studies have shown that the combination of anticoagulation, corticosteroids, and TPE improves survival.[42,49]

Heparin-induced thrombocytopenia

Heparin products are discontinued immediately and the patient is started on a nonheparin anticoagulant such as argatroban, bivalirudin, fondaparinux, or DOACs.[44,46] The choice of anticoagulant depends on the patient's organ function and bleeding risk, the route of administration, and availability of the anticoagulant.[46] If a patient with HIT needs urgent surgery, ASH guideline suggests one of the following:[46]

- Intraoperative anticoagulation with bivalirudin
- Intraoperative heparin after treatment with preoperative and/or intraoperative TPE
- Intraoperative heparin in combination with a potent antiplatelet agent (eg, prostacyclin analogue or tirofiban)

Paroxysmal nocturnal hemoglobinuria

Initiate therapeutic anticoagulation with either UFH or LMWH followed by long-term anticoagulation with VKA.[44,45] Eculizumab, a complement C5 inhibitor, is also initiated to treat PNH.[44,45] Data on the use of DOACs in patients with PNH are limited.[44,45]

Use of direct oral anticoagulants in pediatric patients

There are limited studies on the use of DOACs in pediatric patients. However, a recent clinical trial reported that a body weight–adjusted rivaroxaban regimen showed similar efficacy and safety compared with standard anticoagulation and may be used to treat VTE.[50]

SUMMARY

Coagulopathy in the pediatric setting requires prompt evaluation and directed management. Routine coagulation assays used for the assessment of coagulopathies in pediatric patients need to be interpreted while taking into account the patient's age and being aware of the multiple causes of nonbaseline values in this setting. Patients with congenital coagulopathies often require specialized testing, including von Willebrand panels or individual factor assays. Once identified, recombinant factors or factor concentrates are often used for management. Acquired coagulopathies can develop at any time during childhood. Many of these require treatment with blood components such as FFP or cryoprecipitate, but PCCs may be considered in some settings. Pediatric thrombosis is increasing, largely because of increased awareness and iatrogenic causes. Evaluation and management of thrombosis in pediatric patients is complex and may require involvement of multiple services, including hematology and IR. Initial management usually begins with anticoagulation.[38,47,48] Choice of anticoagulant depends on the patient's clinical status and bleeding risk, and the availability of the drug.[47] When thrombophilia work-up is sent during an acute illness, test results may be abnormal. Therefore, thrombophilia work-up should be repeated when the patient is well.[41]

DISCLOSURE

The authors have nothing to disclose.

REFERENCES

1. Attard C, van der Straaten T, Karlaftis V, et al. Developmental hemostasis: age-specific differences in the levels of hemostatic proteins. J Thromb Haemost 2013;11(10):1850–4.
2. Rodeghiero F, Pabinger I, Ragni M, et al. Fundamentals for a systematic approach to mild and moderate inherited bleeding disorders: an EHA consensus report. Hemasphere 2019;3(5):e286.
3. Chai-Adisaksopha C, Hillis C, Thabane L, et al. A systematic review of definitions and reporting of bleeding outcome measures in haemophilia. Haemophilia 2015; 21(6):731–5.
4. Gilbert L, Paroskie A, Gailani D, et al. Haemophilia A carriers experience reduced health-related quality of life. Haemophilia 2015;21(6):761–5.
5. Armstrong E, Hillarp A. Assay discrepancy in mild haemophilia A. Eur J Haematol Suppl 2014;76:48–50.
6. Duncan EM, Rodgers SE, McRae SJ. Diagnostic testing for mild hemophilia a in patients with discrepant one-stage, two-stage, and chromogenic factor VIII:C assays. Semin Thromb Hemost 2013;39(3):272–82.
7. Kasper CK, Hemophilia of Georgia USA. Protocols for the treatment of haemophilia and von Willebrand disease. Haemophilia 2000;6(Suppl 1):84–93.
8. Girolami A, Scandellari R, Scapin M, et al. Congenital bleeding disorders of the vitamin K-dependent clotting factors. Vitam Horm 2008;78:281–374.
9. Duga S, Salomon O. Congenital factor XI deficiency: an update. Semin Thromb Hemost 2013;39(6):621–31.
10. Santoro C, Di Mauro R, Baldacci E, et al. Bleeding phenotype and correlation with factor XI (FXI) activity in congenital FXI deficiency: results of a retrospective study from a single centre. Haemophilia 2015;21(4):496–501.
11. Michiels JJ, Gadisseur A, Budde U, et al. Characterization, classification, and treatment of von Willebrand diseases: a critical appraisal of the literature and personal experiences. Semin Thromb Hemost 2005;31(5):577–601.
12. Lillicrap D. von Willebrand disease: advances in pathogenetic understanding, diagnosis, and therapy. Hematology Am Soc Hematol Educ Program 2013; 2013:254–60.

13. Nichols WL, Hultin MB, James AH, et al. von Willebrand disease (VWD): evidence-based diagnosis and management guidelines, the national heart, Lung, and blood Institute (NHLBI) Expert panel report (USA). Haemophilia 2008;14(2):171–232.

14. Mensah PK, Gooding R. Surgery in patients with inherited bleeding disorders. Anaesthesia 2015;70(Suppl 1):112–20.e39-40.

15. Levi M, Toh CH, Thachil J, et al. Guidelines for the diagnosis and management of disseminated intravascular coagulation. British Committee for Standards in Haematology. Br J Haematol 2009;145(1):24–33.

16. Soundar EP, Jariwala P, Nguyen TC, et al. Evaluation of the International Society on Thrombosis and Haemostasis and institutional diagnostic criteria of disseminated intravascular coagulation in pediatric patients. Am J Clin Pathol 2013; 139(6):812–6.

17. Rajagopal R, Thachil J, Monagle P. Disseminated intravascular coagulation in paediatrics. Arch Dis Child 2017;102(2):187–93.

18. Sutor AH. Vitamin K deficiency bleeding in infants and children. Semin Thromb Hemost 1995;21(3):317–29.

19. Wicklund BM. Bleeding and clotting disorders in pediatric liver disease. Hematology Am Soc Hematol Educ Program 2011;2011:170–7.

20. Lisman T, Porte RJ. Rebalanced hemostasis in patients with liver disease: evidence and clinical consequences. Blood 2010;116(6):878–85.

21. Lisman T, Leebeek FW, Mosnier LO, et al. Thrombin-activatable fibrinolysis inhibitor deficiency in cirrhosis is not associated with increased plasma fibrinolysis. Gastroenterology 2001;121(1):131–9.

22. Rijken DC, Kock EL, Guimarães AH, et al. Evidence for an enhanced fibrinolytic capacity in cirrhosis as measured with two different global fibrinolysis tests. J Thromb Haemost 2012;10(10):2116–22.

23. Tacke F, Fiedler K, von Depka M, et al. Clinical and prognostic role of plasma coagulation factor XIII activity for bleeding disorders and 6-year survival in patients with chronic liver disease. Liver Int 2006;26(2):173–81.

24. Drebes A, de Vos M, Gill S, et al. Prothrombin complex concentrates for coagulopathy in liver disease: single-center, clinical experience in 105 patients. Hepatol Commun 2019;3(4):513–24.

25. Kwon JO, MacLaren R. Comparison of fresh-frozen plasma, four-factor prothrombin complex concentrates, and recombinant factor VIIa to facilitate procedures in critically Ill patients with coagulopathy from liver disease: a retrospective cohort study. Pharmacotherapy 2016;36(10):1047–54.

26. Liu P, Hum J, Jou J, et al. Transfusion strategies in patients with cirrhosis. Eur J Haematol 2020;104(1):15–25.

27. Hendrickson JE, Shaz BH, Pereira G, et al. Coagulopathy is prevalent and associated with adverse outcomes in transfused pediatric trauma patients. J Pediatr 2012;160(2):204–9.e3.

28. Eckert MJ, Wertin TM, Tyner SD, et al. Tranexamic acid administration to pediatric trauma patients in a combat setting: the pediatric trauma and tranexamic acid study (PED-TRAX). J Trauma Acute Care Surg 2014;77(6):852–8 [discussion: 858].

29. Federici AB, Budde U, Castaman G, et al. Current diagnostic and therapeutic approaches to patients with acquired von Willebrand syndrome: a 2013 update. Semin Thromb Hemost 2013;39(2):191–201.

30. Federici AB. Acquired von Willebrand syndrome associated with hypothyroidism: a mild bleeding disorder to be further investigated. Semin Thromb Hemost 2011; 37(1):35–40.
31. Charlebois J, Rivard G, St-Louis J. Management of acquired von Willebrand syndrome. Transfus Apher Sci 2018;57(6):721–3.
32. Brackmann HH, Schramm W, Oldenburg J, et al. Origins, development, current challenges and future directions with activated prothrombin complex concentrate for the treatment of patients with congenital haemophilia with inhibitors. Hamostaseologie 2020. https://doi.org/10.1055/a-1159-4273.
33. Franchini M, Mannucci PM. Acquired haemophilia A: a 2013 update. Thromb Haemost 2013;110(6):1114–20.
34. Nijenhuis AV, van Bergeijk L, Huijgens PC, et al. Acquired factor XIII deficiency due to an inhibitor: a case report and review of the literature. Haematologica 2004;89(5):ECR14.
35. Gregory TF, Cooper B. Case report of an acquired factor XIII inhibitor: diagnosis and management. Proc (Bayl Univ Med Cent) 2006;19(3):221–3.
36. Lee MT, Nardi MA, Hadzi-Nesic J, et al. Transient hemorrhagic diathesis associated with an inhibitor of prothrombin with lupus anticoagulant in a 1 1/2-year-old girl: report of a case and review of the literature. Am J Hematol 1996;51(4):307–14.
37. Becton DL, Stine KC. Transient lupus anticoagulants associated with hemorrhage rather than thrombosis: the hemorrhagic lupus anticoagulant syndrome. J Pediatr 1997;130(6):998–1000.
38. Mahajerin A, Betensky M, Goldenberg NA. Thrombosis in children: approach to anatomic risks, thrombophilia, prevention, and treatment. Hematol Oncol Clin North Am 2019;33(3):439–53.
39. Haley KM. Neonatal venous thromboembolism. Front Pediatr 2017;5:136.
40. van Ommen CH, Nowak-Göttl U. Inherited thrombophilia in pediatric venous thromboembolic disease: why and who to test. Front Pediatr 2017;5:50.
41. Raffini L. Thrombophilia in children: who to test, how, when, and why? Hematology Am Soc Hematol Educ Program 2008;228–35. https://doi.org/10.1182/asheducation-2008.1.228.
42. Garcia D, Erkan D. Diagnosis and management of the antiphospholipid syndrome. N Engl J Med 2018;379(13):1290.
43. Wincup C, Ioannou Y. The differences between childhood and adult onset antiphospholipid syndrome. Front Pediatr 2018;6:362.
44. Skeith L. Anticoagulating patients with high-risk acquired thrombophilias. Blood 2018;132(21):2219–29.
45. Patriquin CJ, Kiss T, Caplan S, et al. How we treat paroxysmal nocturnal hemoglobinuria: a consensus statement of the Canadian PNH Network and review of the national registry. Eur J Haematol 2019;102(1):36–52.
46. Cuker A, Arepally GM, Chong BH, et al. American Society of Hematology 2018 guidelines for management of venous thromboembolism: heparin-induced thrombocytopenia. Blood Adv 2018;2(22):3360–92.
47. Monagle P, Cuello CA, Augustine C, et al. American Society of Hematology 2018 Guidelines for management of venous thromboembolism: treatment of pediatric venous thromboembolism. Blood Adv 2018;2(22):3292–316.
48. Monagle P, Chan AKC, Goldenberg NA, et al. Antithrombotic therapy in neonates and children: Antithrombotic therapy and prevention of thrombosis, 9th ed:

American College of chest Physicians evidence-based clinical Practice guide-lines. Chest 2012;141(2 Suppl):e737S–801S.

49. Carmi O, Berla M, Shoenfeld Y, et al. Diagnosis and management of catastrophic antiphospholipid syndrome. Expert Rev Hematol 2017;10(4):365–74.

50. Young G, Lensing AWA, Monagle P, et al. Rivaroxaban for treatment of pediatric venous thromboembolism. An Einstein-Jr phase 3 dose-exposure-response eval-uation. J Thromb Haemost 2020;18(7):1672–85.

Transfusion and Cellular Therapy in Pediatric Sickle Cell Disease

Yan Zheng, MD, PhD[a], Stella T. Chou, MD[b],*

KEYWORDS

- Sickle cell disease • Red blood cell transfusion • Alloimmunization • Iron overload
- Hematopoietic stem cell transplant • Apheresis • Plerixafor

KEY POINTS

- Red blood cell (RBC) transfusion is a mainstay treatment of acute and chronic complications of sickle cell disease (SCD). Prophylactic transfusion with Rh (C, E or C/c, E/e) and K-matched RBCs is recommended to prevent RBC alloimmunization. Iron status should be closely monitored in patients receiving chronic transfusion.
- Matched sibling donor hematopoietic stem cell transplant (HSCT) is a treatment option for patients with SCD. Platelets should be maintained at greater than or equal to $50 \times 10^3/\mu L$ and hemoglobin 9 to 11 g/dL in the peritransplant period. RBC and human leukocyte antigen alloimmunization are strongly associated with increased transfusion demands.
- Autologous HSCT with gene-corrected hematopoietic stem cells (HSCs) for SCD requires a large number of cells. Plerixafor enables rapid and efficient HSC mobilization with minimal toxicity. Hydroxyurea cessation and optimized HSC leukocytapheresis collection increase the HSC yield.

TRANSFUSION MANAGEMENT OF SICKLE CELL DISEASE

Red blood cell (RBC) transfusion is an essential treatment of sickle cell disease (SCD), with more than 50% of affected children receiving at least 1 transfusion.[1] RBC transfusion improves blood oxygen delivery by reducing the percentage of hemoglobin S (HbS%) and blood viscosity. Transfusion continues to be a common therapy for prevention and management of acute and chronic complications of SCD.[2–4]

Funding: The authors acknowledge support from the American Lebanese Syrian Associated Charities (Y. Zheng), National Blood Foundation Early-Stage Investigator's Award (Y. Zheng), and the National Institutes of Health/National Heart Lung Blood Institute HL134696 and HL147879-01 (S.T. Chou).

a Department of Pathology, St. Jude Children's Research Hospital, MS 342, 262 Danny Thomas Place, Memphis, TN 38105, USA; b Department of Pediatrics, The Children's Hospital of Philadelphia, University of Pennsylvania School of Medicine, 3615 Civic Center Boulevard, Abramson Research Center Room 316D, Philadelphia, PA 19010, USA
* Corresponding author.
E-mail address: chous@email.chop.edu

Clin Lab Med 41 (2021) 101–119
https://doi.org/10.1016/j.cll.2020.10.007
0272-2712/21/© 2020 Elsevier Inc. All rights reserved.

Red Blood Cell Transfusion Method

RBCs can be infused via simple transfusion or by red blood cell exchange (RBCX).[5] A comparison of the different transfusion methods is summarized in **Table 1**. Simple transfusion can be administered via peripheral access and does not require specialized devices or trained personnel. Chronic simple transfusion inevitably leads to iron overload, and, thus, initiation of iron chelation therapy is recommended after 1 to 2 years of transfusions and when the serum ferritin level exceeds 1000 ng/mL on 2 occasions or the liver iron content is greater than 3 mg/g dry weight.[6] To avoid potential blood hyperviscosity, simple transfusion should only increase the hemoglobin level (Hb) to 10 to 11 g/dL, particularly when HbS% is greater than 50%.

RBCX replaces RBCs containing hemoglobin S (HbS) with healthy donor cells, thereby reducing HbS% with minimal effects on blood viscosity, fluid balance, and iron burden. RBCX is indicated for patients with high pretransfusion Hb levels (ie, Hb>9–10 g/dL), for specific complications including acute ischemic stroke, for patients with cardiac disease who are unable to tolerate the added volume of a simple transfusion, and for individuals with iron overload and unable to iron chelate. For RBCX, a target HbS% of less than or equal to 30% is often used to prevent and manage most SCD-associated complications.[7,8] Although RBCX increases donor unit exposures, it does not seem to increase the risk of alloimmunization.[9] RBCX can be performed by manual RBCX, automated RBCX, and automated RBCX with isovolemic hemodilution (IHD). Manual RBCX sequentially removes patient blood and infuses donor RBCs, and typically requires 2 to 8 hours to complete. Automated RBCX can reach target hematocrit (Hct) and HbS% levels in 1 to 3 hours and can maintain isovolemia to support hemodynamic stability. Automated RBCX requires apheresis devices and trained staff, which may not be available in small community centers. For pediatric patients with low body weight, apheresis devices should be primed with donor RBCs to prevent substantial intraprocedure volume shifts and acute anemia caused by the large extracorporeal volume of the apheresis devices for these patients. Central venous access is often required for automated RBCX to provide sufficient venous access for the rapid blood flow rates and high negative pressure in the withdrawal line. For patients requiring chronic transfusion therapy, automated RBCX is recommended rather than simple transfusion or manual RBCX if possible.[2] Automated RBCX-IHD includes an initial phase of IHD or depletion in which patient

Table 1 Comparison of blood transfusion method			
	Simple Transfusion	**Manual RBCX**	**Automated RBCX**
Specialized instrument	No	No	Yes
Trained personnel	No	Yes	Yes
Vascular access	Peripheral	Central venous catheter might be required	Central venous catheter might be required
RBC exposure	Fewest	Intermediate	Highest
Hyperviscosity	High risk[a]	Intermediate risk[a]	Minimal risk
Fluid balance	Potential fluid overload	Minimal volume shifts	Isovolemic
Iron overload	Inevitable	Intermediate risk	Minimal risk

[a] Minimized by avoiding posttransfusion hemoglobin level greater than 11 g/dL.

blood is replaced by saline or 5% albumin instead of donor RBCs. This technique may slightly decrease the donor unit requirement, compared with conventional automated RBCX, to reach the same target HbS% level. Although RBCX-IHD maintains isovolemia, saline/or albumin replacement acutely decreases the patient's Hct. Therefore, RBCX-IHD is not recommended for patients with acute complications (ie, stroke or acute chest syndrome) or for those with severe central nervous system disease, vasculopathy, or cardiopulmonary disease, in which further anemia during the IHD phase may be detrimental.[2] It is recommended not to decrease the Hct to less than 21% and/or more than 20% from the patient's baseline.[2] For patients experiencing hypotension during the depletion phase, 5% albumin can be used as a replacement fluid.

Indications for Red Blood Cell Transfusion

RBC transfusion is a mainstay treatment of various complications of SCD (**Table 2**). The benefit of chronic transfusion therapy is well established for preventing primary and secondary strokes, and recurrent silent cerebral infarctions (SCIs). Transfusion can correct acute anemia in aplastic crises and acute splenic and hepatic sequestration, and can reduce HbS% in acute chest syndrome (ACS), acute stroke, acute multiorgan failure, and acute intrahepatic cholestasis. Transfusion also decreases SCD-associated complications in patients undergoing surgery and during pregnancy. Transfusion is not recommended for patients with steady-state anemia, uncomplicated painful vaso-occlusive crisis (VOC), priapism, leg ulcers, and nonsurgically managed avascular necrosis. For patients with recurrent ACS, recurrent VOC, pulmonary hypertension, and uncomplicated pregnancy, the benefit of transfusion is not established; therefore, transfusion therapy should be considered on a case-by-case basis.

Neurologic complications

Approximately 11% of individuals with SCD are estimated to experience overt strokes by age 20 years.[10] Children with SCD who are at risk for stroke can be identified by abnormally high blood flow velocity on transcranial Doppler ultrasonography (TCD).[11] In the Stroke Prevention in Sickle Cell Anemia (STOP 1) trial, chronic transfusion to maintain HbS% less than 30% reduced the incidence of initial strokes in children with abnormal TCD findings by 92%.[12] The STOP 2 trial supported the use of chronic transfusion indefinitely, because discontinuation after 30 months resulted in an increased rate of abnormal TCD conversion and stroke.[13] Most recently, the TCD with Transfusions Changing to Hydroxyurea (TWiTCH) trial showed that hydroxyurea is not inferior to chronic transfusion for primary stoke prevention by reducing TCD velocities in children with abnormal TCDs.[14] Given the burden and potential side effects of chronic transfusion therapy, the ability to prevent stroke with hydroxyurea is a major advance.

Chronic transfusion is the standard of care for secondary stroke prevention. Up to 90% of patients with a stroke may experience a recurrence without therapeutic intervention, and the risk of secondary stroke decreases to ~20% with chronic transfusion therapy that maintains a HbS% less than 30%.[15–17] Indefinite transfusion therapy is recommended because the Stroke With Transfusions Changing to Hydroxyurea (SWiTCH) trial was closed because of statistical futility on the composite end point of iron overload resolution and stroke prevention. At time of study closure, 10% of patients treated with hydroxyurea and phlebotomy had experienced a second stroke, compared with no patients receiving chronic transfusion therapy.[18]

SCIs are more common than overt stroke, and 25% of children with SCD experience SCIs.[19,20] SCIs are associated with an increased risk of new or enlarged SCIs, overt

Table 2
Indications for transfusion in patients with sickle cell disease

Condition	Transfusion Indication	Transfusion Method
Acute ischemic stroke	Accepted	Exchange transfusion preferred
Primary stroke prevention	Accepted	Chronic simple or exchange transfusion
Secondary stroke prevention	Accepted	Chronic simple or exchange transfusion
Acute chest syndrome, severe[a]	Accepted	Exchange transfusion preferred
Acute chest syndrome, moderate	Accepted	Simple or exchange transfusion
Acute splenic sequestration	Accepted	Simple transfusion
Acute splenic sequestration, recurrent	Accepted	Chronic simple transfusion (before splenectomy)
Preoperative (surgeries requiring general anesthesia and lasting >1 h)	Accepted	Simple or exchange transfusion[b]
Transient aplastic crisis	Accepted	Simple transfusion
Acute multiorgan failure	Accepted	Simple or exchange transfusion
Acute hepatic sequestration	Accepted	Simple or exchange transfusion
Acute intrahepatic cholestasis	Accepted	Simple or exchange transfusion
Pregnancy, complicated[c]	Accepted	Prophylactic simple or exchange transfusion
Acute chest syndrome, recurrent	Controversial	Chronic simple or exchange transfusion
Vaso-occlusive crisis, recurrent	Controversial	Chronic simple or exchange transfusion
Pulmonary hypertension	Controversial	Chronic simple or exchange transfusion
Vaso-occlusive crisis, uncomplicated	Not indicated	NA
Priapism	Not indicated	NA
Leg ulcers	Not indicated	NA
Avascular necrosis, nonsurgically managed	Not indicated	NA
Pregnancy, uncomplicated	Unknown benefit	NA

Abbreviation: NA, not available.
    [a] Severe acute chest syndrome, usually considered with rapidly declining hemoglobin levels, severe hypoxia (Spo_2 ≤94% or considerably below patient baseline), and/or requiring invasive respiratory support.
    [b] Exchange transfusion when pretransfusion hemoglobin level is greater than 9 to 10 g/dL, which precludes administration of simple transfusion, or for high-risk surgery (eg, neurosurgery).
    [c] Pregnant women with a history of severe or frequent SCD-related complications before the current pregnancy, onset of SCD-related complications during current pregnancy, or high-risk pregnancy.

stroke, low intelligence quotient (IQ), and poor academic performance.[20–22] The Silent Cerebral Infarct Multi-Center Clinical Trial (SIT) showed that chronic transfusion therapy decreased the incidence of recurrent SCIs by 58% (14% in the observation group compared with 6% in the transfusion group).[23] Given the high incidence of SCIs in children with SCD, the resources needed to provide chronic transfusion therapy to this entire group would be considerable, and thus chronic transfusion therapy is usually considered for those at highest risk (ie, magnetic resonance angiography–defined vasculopathy, poor school performance). The efficacy of hydroxyurea for preventing recurrent SCIs is yet to be determined.

Acute chest syndrome

ACS is the leading cause of death and second most common cause of hospitalization for patients with SCD.[24] The clinical presentation of ACS varies from fever, cough, chest pain, and mild dyspnea to severe hypoxia requiring ventilation, and even death.[25] RBC transfusion is often used to treat moderate and severe ACS, in addition to antimicrobial and respiratory support.[26–28] No established clinical or laboratory criteria are available to define the severity of ACS or to identify patients with poor prognosis. Severe ACS is usually considered in patients with rapidly declining Hb levels, significant hypoxia ($SpO_2 \leq 94\%$ or considerably less than patient baseline), and/or requiring invasive respiratory support.[2] RBCX is recommended rather than simple transfusion for severe ACS management.[2] However, if a significant delay is expected while mobilizing blood and apheresis personnel, simple transfusion should be administered in the interim to patients with Hb levels less than 9 g/dL. There is insufficient evidence to support RBCX rather than simple transfusion for moderate ACS, so either is appropriate.[2] However, RBCX should be considered for patients with rapidly progressive ACS, those who do not respond to simple transfusion, or those with pretransfusion Hb levels greater than or equal to 9 to 10 g/dL that preclude simple transfusion. Recurrent ACS occurs in 44% of patients with SCD,[29] for which the primary treatment is hydroxyurea.[3] Chronic transfusion reduces the incidence of ACS and subsequent hospitalizations, so should be considered if hydroxyurea is ineffective or contraindicated.[22,23,30]

Preoperative transfusion support

Patients with SCD may experience ACS, painful VOC, and other postoperative complications, particularly for patients with low preoperative Hb levels (<9 g/dL), severe SCD genotypes (ie, Hemoglobin SS or Hemoglobin Sβ° thalassemia) or phenotypes, and those receiving high-risk surgery (cardiac and neurosurgery). The Transfusion Alternatives Preoperatively in Sickle Cell Disease (TAPS) trial showed that preoperative transfusion to increase Hb levels to 10 g/dL reduces the risk of overall perioperative complications, particularly ACS, in patients undergoing low-risk to moderate-risk surgeries.[31] Patients receiving aggressive preoperative transfusion to reach a Hb level of 10 g/dL and HbS% less than 30% experience a similar number of perioperative complications to those having conservative preoperative transfusion to only increase Hb levels to 10 g/dL (with no specific target HbS%).[32] Furthermore, preoperative transfusion does not improve hospital stay duration, readmission rate, or mortality of patients with SCD.[31] Hence, preoperative transfusions to increase Hb levels to 10 g/dL (with no specific target HbS%) are recommended for patients with SCD requiring surgery with general anesthesia and lasting greater than 1 hour.[2] RBCX should be considered for patients with high baseline Hb levels (>9–10 g/dL) or undergoing high-risk surgery.

Complications of Red Blood Cell Transfusion

Alloimmunization

Non-ABO antigen RBC alloimmunization remains a significant complication of transfusion. It may also lead to difficulty identifying compatible units and transfusion delays for acute complications of SCD, and may affect the ability to provide transfusion support for hematopoietic stem cell transplant (HSCT) and surgeries with a high risk of blood loss. Alloimmunization can lead to life-threatening reactions that reduce the survival of patients with SCD.[33,34]

Alloimmunization increases the risk of hemolytic transfusion reactions, both acute and delayed. Delayed hemolytic transfusion reactions (DHTRs) occur in 4% to 16% of transfused patients with SCD. DHTRs are classically caused by evanescent alloantibodies, which are undetectable at the time of transfusion, but appear on reexposure to the offending RBC antigens.[35] Patients usually present within 7 to 10 days (and up to 28 days) from the last transfusion with signs and symptoms of anemia and hemolysis, including fatigue, jaundice, hemoglobinuria, fever, and/or pain. Often the direct antiglobulin test (DAT) is positive, and the evanescent alloantibodies are identified, but not always. When a new antibody is identified, the patient's Hb, reticulocyte count, and HbS% should be obtained to evaluate for laboratory evidence suggestive of hemolysis. High clinical suspicion and monitoring for DHTRs are warranted, because they may be more common than is appreciated in patients with SCD and are sometimes clinically subtle.[36] Rarely, hyperhemolysis syndrome occurs, in which both transfused and endogenous RBCs are hemolyzed, leading to severe and potentially lethal anemia.[37] The DAT is often negative in hyperhemolysis syndrome, and no antibody specificity is identified. Patients should be managed with supportive treatment (oxygen and erythropoietin) and immunosuppressive therapy. Intravenous immunoglobulin and/or steroids should be initiated promptly, whereas eculizumab may be considered for those unresponsive to first-line agents.[2] Transfusion is contraindicated in hyperhemolysis syndrome unless the anemia is life threatening. If transfusion is warranted, extended-matched (C/c, E/e, K, Jk^a/Jk^b, Fy^a/Fy^b, S/s) RBCs should be considered.[2] For patients requiring transfusion in the following weeks to months (ie, chronic transfusion for stroke prophylaxis), rituximab may be considered, particularly if no specific antibody is identified.

The prevalence and rate of alloimmunization are higher in patients with SCD than in patients with other diseases.[38] Although alloimmunization prevalence can approach 50% in chronically transfused individuals, the rate of alloimmunization is approximately 0.3 to 0.5 alloantibodies per 100 units transfused with Rh-matched and K-matched transfusion regardless of chronic versus episodic transfusion.[23,39–42] Alloimmunization risk is associated with transfusion burden, RBC antigen differences between patients of African descent and white blood donors, patient immune responses, and inflammatory status when receiving transfusion.[39,43,44]

Alloantibodies commonly identified in patients with SCD include antibodies against Rh (D, C/c, E/e), K, Duffy (Fy^a, Fy^b), Kidd (Jk^a, Jk^b), and S, in part because of the discrepant antigen expression in patients of primarily African ethnicity compared with most donors with European background in the United States.[45] To avoid alloimmunization, prophylactic antigen matching with Rh (C, E, or C/c, E/e) and K-matched RBCs is recommended.[2–4] Extended RBC antigen matching to also include Duffy, Kidd, and S antigens can provide further protection from alloimmunization,[46] but identifying adequate matched units would be challenging.[47,48]

Prophylactic antigen matching requires blood group antigen information. An extended antigen profile (ie, C/c, E/e, K, Jka/Jkb, Fya/Fyb, M/N, and S/s at minimum) is preferred and should be obtained at the earliest opportunity, ideally before the first transfusion.[2] Knowledge of the antigen profile also assists antibody identification and additional antigen matching in alloimmunized patients. An RBC antigen genotype is preferred to a serologic phenotype because it provides additional information and increased accuracy for Fy^b and Rh antigen matching.[2] Patients with mutations in the transcription factor GATA-1 binding site of the *ACKR1/DARC* gene encoding Fy antigens do not express Fy^b on RBCs.[49] These patients are not at risk of forming anti-Fy^b because Fy^b is expressed in other tissues and can thereby safely receive Fy^b+ RBCs. RBC genotyping can also identify variant Rh antigens that are common in African-descended individuals and contribute to Rh alloimmunization despite serologic Rh antigen matching.[40,50,51] Variant Rh antigens, caused by extensive single nucleotide polymorphisms and genetic rearrangements of *RH* genes, differ from conventional Rh antigens with loss of common Rh epitopes and/or expression of new Rh epitopes. Patients may become Rh alloimmunized when exposed to Rh antigens that are absent on their own RBCs. More than 50 Rh variant antigens and more than 500 *RH* variant alleles have been described, with the number of newly identified alleles continuing to increase.[52,53] Although serologic Rh antigen matching decreases Rh alloimmunization, *RH* genotype matching between patients and blood donors is likely needed to eliminate Rh alloantibody formation.[54]

Iron overload

Patients receiving chronic simple transfusion and those who undergo RBCX but require an increase in their end procedure Hct accumulate iron stores. Free iron accumulates in the liver, heart, and endocrine system, resulting in organ dysfunction. Because SCD-associated inflammation promotes iron retention in the reticuloendothelial system, the liver is the most commonly affected organ.[55] Cardiac iron overload is uncommon for patients with SCD and typically occurs in a subgroup of patients with exceedingly high iron levels over a prolonged period of time.[56–58]

Iron burden can be evaluated by serum ferritin levels, and liver and cardiac MRI. Serum ferritin levels can be readily and frequently obtained and are a convenient option for monitoring iron burden over time.[59] However, serum ferritin levels increase with SCD-associated inflammation and may not be a reliable marker for total-body iron burden. Liver iron content (LIC) is a good indicator of total-body iron burden and was traditionally assessed by liver biopsy.[60,61] LIC measured by MRI (R2, T2*, or R2*) correlates well with liver biopsy results and has become the primary screening tool for iron overload.[62,63] LIC should be screened by MRI every 1 to 2 years for patients on chronic transfusion therapy and/or with a serum iron level greater than or equal to 1000 ng/mL.[2] Cardiac iron overload is uncommon for patients with SCD, and thus routine cardiac iron content screening by T2* MRI is not required unless a history of poor iron control, cardiac dysfunction, or other end-organ damage is identified.[2]

Iron chelation therapy (ie, deferoxamine and deferasirox) can maintain a negative or neutral iron balance to prevent hemosiderosis. The ferritin trend and liver R2* measurements of iron accumulation are used to titrate iron chelation regimens. For patients with severe iron overload, combination iron chelation can be used, or iron chelation therapy may be combined with RBCX.

ALLOGENEIC HEMATOPOIETIC STEM CELL TRANSPLANT AND TRANSFUSION SUPPORT

HSCT as a curative therapy for SCD was first reported in 1984, in which a patient with SCD received HSCT for leukemia and both disorders were cured.[64] Since then, various conditioning regimens, such as myeloablative, reduced-intensity, and non-myeloablative regimens, and different hematopoietic stem cell (HSC) sources, including human leukocyte antigen (HLA)–matched sibling donors, unrelated HLA-matched donors, umbilical cord blood, and haploidentical-related donors, have been examined in multiple clinical trials. Matched sibling donor HSCT, with a high overall survival rate (>90%), low incidence of graft rejection (<3%), and chronic graft-versus-host disease (GVHD; <15%), has evolved into a curative treatment option for pediatric patients with SCD with fully matched sibling donors.[65,66] Pediatric patients with less SCD-associated end-organ damage than adult patients are more likely to tolerate intense conditioning regimens. Transfusion support for patients with SCD undergoing HSCT requires specific considerations because of the unique clinical characteristics of SCD and prevalence of RBC and HLA alloimmunization in this patient population.

Transfusion Support

Reducing the HbS% to less than 30% by simple transfusion or RBCX for months or just before the start of HSCT conditioning has become common practice. In a murine model of SCD, SCD-associated inflammation and hypoxia lead to vascular tortuosity and sinusoidal stasis in bone marrow, which are reversed by chronic transfusion therapy.[67] This observation suggests that pre-HSCT blood transfusions can be beneficial by altering the marrow environment to improve engraftment. This benefit must be weighed against the risk of RBC and HLA alloimmunization and other transfusion reactions. Therefore, the number and duration of pre-HSCT transfusions should be individualized.

During the peri-HSCT period, patients with SCD are at increased risk of neurovascular complications, including intracranial hemorrhage, seizure, and posterior reversible encephalopathy syndrome (PRES).[68] The transfusion threshold for platelets is less than $50 \times 10^3/\mu L$ to prevent intracranial hemorrhage, and maintenance of platelet counts above this transfusion threshold is particularly important for patients with a history of stroke. Hb should be maintained between 9 and 11 g/dL to prevent both anemia and hyperviscosity. The risk of PRES and seizures can be further decreased by close monitoring and control of electrolytes and blood pressure.

Blood products selected for patients with SCD undergoing HSCT should meet certain criteria. All blood products should be irradiated and leukoreduced. Irradiation prevents transfusion-associated GVHD. Leukoreduction decreases febrile nonhemolytic transfusion reactions, HLA sensitization, and transmission of infectious diseases carried in white blood cells (eg, cytomegalovirus). Patients with SCD should receive HbS-negative RBC units, ideally stored for less than 14 to 21 days to maximize in vivo circulatory half-life. Units should be prophylactically matched for Rh (C, E, or C/c, E/e) and K antigens of the patients, and lacking antigens against which the patient has previously formed alloantibodies. Some transfusion services extend the matching to Fy^a/Fy^b, Jk^a/Jk^b and S antigens, particularly if a patient is heavily alloimmunized.

ABO Incompatibility as a Special Consideration

Major ABO incompatibility refers to the presence of natural anti-A and/or anti-B antibodies in recipients against donor A and/or B blood group antigens. Major ABO incompatibility can cause (1) acute intravascular hemolysis of donor RBCs present in HSC products on infusion; and (2) chronic destruction of donor erythrocyte precursors, leading to delayed RBC engraftment (DRE) and even pure RBC aplasia (PRCA).[69] Acute hemolysis is rare when HSC products are collected by apheresis because these products typically contain 2% to 5% RBCs and a total RBC volume of less than 20 mL.[8] In contrast, HSC products collected by bone marrow harvest have an increased risk caused by a high RBC content of 25% to 35%. Acute hemolytic transfusion reaction can be minimized by RBC reduction during HSC product processing by automatic cell processors, hydroxyethyl starch sedimentation, or Ficoll-Paque density gradient separation.[69] General practice is to not exceed 0.3 to 0.4 mL/kg or a total of 10 to 30 mL of RBCs for pediatric patients receiving an HSC product with ABO incompatibility.[70]

Recipient ABO antibodies can persist for many months causing DRE and PRCA, leading to prolonged transfusion dependence after HSCT. The primary source of ABO antibodies is recipient plasma cells.[71] Patients undergoing nonmyeloablative and reduced-intensity HSCT are at particular risk because their own plasma cells are more likely to persist. PRCA is treated with erythropoietin, rapid tapering of immunosuppressants, and supportive transfusions. Although therapeutic plasma exchange may theoretically improve PRCA by removing incompatible ABO antibodies, it is not recommended because of its inability to remove antibody-producing recipient plasma cells.[72]

Minor ABO incompatibility refers to the presence of natural anti-A and/or anti-B antibodies in donors against recipient A and/or B blood group antigens. Minor ABO incompatibility can cause transient and usually self-limited hemolysis of recipient RBCs during infusion, which can be avoided by plasma reduction of HSC products to less than 200 to 300 mL or 5 mL/kg.[69,70] In addition, clinically severe and possibly fatal hemolysis can occur 5 to 16 days after HSCT caused by passenger lymphocyte syndrome, in which donor lymphocytes in grafts produce antibodies against recipient RBCs after sensitization to recipient antigens.[69] In severe cases, RBCX can be used to replace recipient RBCs with donor-compatible RBCs.

To support ABO incompatible HSCT, RBC and plasma-rich components compatible with both donors and recipients are selected.[69] Specifically, for ABO major incompatible HSCT (eg, blood type O recipients transplanted with blood type A donor), RBCs compatible with both donors and recipients are transfused (blood type O in this case). For ABO minor incompatible HSCT (eg, blood type A recipient transplanted with blood type O donor), plasma-rich components compatible with both donors and recipients are chosen (blood types A and AB in this case).

Red Blood Cell and Human Leukocyte Antigen Alloimmunization as a Special Consideration

Patients with SCD often require more transfusion support in the peri-HSCT period compared with patients with other disorders, and their transfusion requirements vary considerably. In 1 study, a median of 7 RBC transfusions (range, 3–15) and 13.5 platelet transfusions (range, 4–48) per patient were administered before reaching transfusion independence.[73] The increased transfusion demands may be caused by the high prophylactic transfusion thresholds and the high prevalence of RBC and/or HLA alloimmunization in this patient population.

Red blood cell alloimmunization
RBC alloimmunization is common in patients with SCD undergoing HSCT, with approximately 31% to 36% of patients having a history of RBC alloimmunization.[74,75] RBC alloimmunization is strongly associated with increased RBC transfusion demands (7 units for RBC-alloimmunized patients vs 4 units for nonalloimmunized patients in the first 45 days after HSCT).[75] For alloimmunized recipients with antibodies against donor RBC antigens, recipient plasma cells that have survived the conditioning regimens may continue to produce donor-specific RBC antibodies resulting in DRE or PRCA. Notably, 1 study found that patients who were alloimmunized but lacked antibodies specific to their donor RBC antigens also required more transfusions (6.5 units for RBC-alloimmunized patients vs 4 units for RBC-nonalloimmunized patients in the first 45 days after HSCT).[75] Because these patients were treated with nonmyeloablative conditioning regimens, their residual immune responses may have removed donor and/or transfused RBCs in an antibody-independent manner. For alloimmunized patients, HSC donor RBC antigen

profiles should be considered when selecting from equivalent HLA-matched donors, and extended antigen-matched RBCs may be indicated for select patients. Advance communication between the transplant and transfusion services can be helpful for both HSC donor selection and peri-HSCT transfusion support.

Human leukocyte antigen alloimmunization

Patients with SCD managed with chronic transfusion therapy are at risk for HLA alloimmunization. Approximately 30% of patients undergoing HSCT have HLA class I antibodies.[74,76] Because HLA class I antigens are present on platelets and crossmatch-compatible or HLA-matched platelets are not routinely administered, HLA class I alloimmunization can lead to poor posttransfusion platelet increments or platelet refractoriness. Specifically, platelet refractoriness is defined as 1-hour posttransfusion corrected count increments less than 5000 to 7000/μL ([platelet increment (μL) × body surface area (m^2)]/[number of single platelet units × 3]). In limited studies of pediatric patients with SCD undergoing HLA-matched HSCT, those with HLA class I antibodies required nearly twice as many platelet transfusions (2.5–19 units for HLA alloimmunized vs 1–7.5 units for HLA nonalloimmunized in the first 45 days after HSCT).[74,76] High platelet transfusion burden is associated with adverse outcomes in the context of HSCT and various transfusion reactions, in particular pulmonary complications.[77,78] HLA antibody screening before HSCT for patients on chronic transfusion is recommended to identify patients at risk for platelet refractoriness and to estimate the potential need for crossmatch-compatible or HLA-matched platelets.

COMPLICATIONS OF PERI-HSCT RED BLOOD CELL TRANSFUSION
Red Blood Cell Alloimmunization

Patients with SCD remain at risk for new RBC alloantibody formation during the peri-HSCT period, which is more likely with nonmyeloablative HSCT. Nonmyeloablative conditioning regimens often result in mixed chimerism of donor-derived and recipient-derived RBCs and immune cells. Residual recipient immune cells can form antibodies against donor RBC antigens, causing hemolysis of donor RBCs and DRE or PRCA. Donor-derived immune cells can become immunized to recipient RBC antigens, resulting in hemolysis. Furthermore, both donor- and recipient-derived immune cells can form antibodies against transfused RBCs. In a study of 61 patients undergoing nonmyeloablative HLA-matched or haploidentical HSCT, 6 patients formed 11 new RBC alloantibodies and 2 autoantibodies.[75] Three of the alloantibodies were acquired during peri-HSCT transfusions, and incompatible with either donor or recipient antigens. Most of the new antibodies were detected within 30 days of HSCT; the median time to first detection was 17 days. Two patients experienced acute hemolysis and 3 patients had DRE with severe anemia. Pretransplant extended RBC antigen phenotyping or genotyping of patients and donors can identify potential mismatches, and prophylactic extended RBC matching (beyond Rh and Kell) can be considered but may not be feasible because of donor availability.

AUTOLOGOUS HEMATOPOIETIC STEM CELL TRANSPLANT AND TRANSFUSION SUPPORT

Allogeneic HSCT from HLA-matched sibling donors is an established curative therapy for SCD, but many patients lack an unaffected HLA-matched sibling donor. Identifying unrelated HLA-matched donors is also challenging because of the low number of African-descended individuals in bone marrow donor registries.[79] Clinical trials using alternative donor options, including umbilical cord blood or haploidentical-related donors, have had encouraging results but are also associated with a high incidence of graft rejection and GVHD.[80–83] Autologous HSC gene therapy provides a novel approach with the potential to be available to all patients and to avoid many complications or toxicities associated with allogeneic HSCT. Many gene editing strategies are currently under investigation, including correction of SCD-causing mutations, overexpression of healthy or modified β^A-like globin gene, and induction of fetal globin expression to outcompete sickle β globin during Hb assembly.[84,85] Multiple phase I/II clinical trials are ongoing and the first patient who received a modified β^A-globin gene encoding an antisickling variant (β^{A87}Thr:Gln [β^{A-T87Q}]) in 2014 achieved complete clinical remission.[86]

A large number of HSCs, approximately 10×10^6/kg to 15×10^6/kg, are required for most gene therapies for SCD.[84] HSCs are preferentially collected from peripheral blood via leukocytapheresis because cells harvested by bone marrow aspiration require general anesthesia, require at least 2 to 4 procedures to obtain an adequate HSC number, and are associated with an increased risk of complications in patients with SCD. Bone marrow mobilization is needed for adequate HSC collection by leukocytapheresis. Granulocyte colony-stimulating factor is contraindicated in patients with SCD because of severe adverse events, such as VOC, ACS, massive splenomegaly, and even death.[87–89] Plerixafor, a CXCR4 (C-X-C chemokine receptor type 4) antagonist, can enable rapid and efficient HSC mobilization with minimal toxicity in patients with SCD (**Table 3**).[90–93] Plerixafor reversibly blocks interaction between CXCR4 on HSCs and stromal-derived factor-1α (SDF-1α) in bone marrow niche,[94] which induces rapid release of HSCs from bone marrow into the peripheral circulation, with peripheral blood cluster of differentiation (CD) 34^+ cell counts peaking as early as 3 to 6 hours after administration. Plerixafor-mobilized HSCs contain a high percentage of long-term repopulating HSCs (CD34^{high}/CD90$^+$/CD45RA$^-$), which are amenable to genetic modification.[91,93,95] Adverse events associated with plerixafor mobilization are mild and limited to VOC that resolves with medical therapy.[90–93] Approximately 3×10^6 to 6×10^6 CD34$^+$ cells per kilogram can be obtained in a single leukocytapheresis collection; therefore, 2 to 3 collections with plerixafor mobilization are typically required to obtain sufficient HSCs for gene therapy.[90,91,93] Additional agents are currently being investigated,[84] including GROβ, a CXCR2 agonist that efficiently mobilizes highly engraftable long-term repopulating HSCs alone or synergistically with plerixafor.[96,97]

HSC yields from leukocytapheresis collections vary considerably among patients, which can be attributed to multiple factors, including hydroxyurea treatment and the unique characteristics of SCD-derived HSCs. Hydroxyurea suppresses bone marrow hematopoiesis, reducing CD34$^+$ cell numbers in the bone marrow and peripheral blood at steady state and on mobilization.[98,99] Hydroxyurea is typically discontinued in the months before HSC collection and replaced by simple RBC transfusion or RBCX.[91,93] The optimal Hb and HbS% levels and duration of transfusions before marrow mobilization are unknown, but Hb levels of 10 g/dL and/or HbS% less than 30% are parameters used by several recent and ongoing clinical trials.[90,91,93]

Despite successful bone marrow mobilization, patients with SCD have lower HSC collection efficiency and yield than do other patients using standard leukocytapheresis.[84,100] SCD-associated inflammation is thought to alter the physical properties of HSCs, resulting in adhesion of the HSCs to other cells. Consequently, SCD-derived HSCs may migrate to a deeper layer during centrifugation and thereby fail to be collected with standard leukocytapheresis techniques. Deeper interface collection improves HSC collection efficiency and yield[90,93] but increases RBC contamination of

Table 3
Plerixafor hematopoietic stem cell mobilization in patients with sickle cell disease

Study	Plerixafor Dose (µg/kg)	Patients (N)	Patient Age (y)	Male (%)	Patients on HU (N)	Patients with Transfusions Before Plerixafor (N)	Preplerixafor HbS (%)	Peak CD34 Count (/µL)	Product Hct (%)	CD34+ Cell Yield (×10^6/kg)	Adverse Events
Uchida et al,[93] 2020	240	15	29[a] (20–50)	47	11	15	27 (15.1–37.7)	52 (9–183)	4.5 (2.7–7.5)	6.3 (2.2–12.0)	5[c]
Lagresle-Peyrou et al,[91] 2018	240	3	20 (19–21)	100	1	3	<30	>80	5.8 (4.8–8.2)	4.6 (4.5–5.8)	0
Esrick et al,[90] 2018	180	3	26 (19–30)	100	0	3	9.9 (5.5–13.3)	36 (31–65)	5.6 (3.7–17)	0.616 (0.069–1.2)	0
	240	3	25 (25–38)	100	0	3	9.2 (6.9–21.4)	156 (27–290)	11.7 (10.5–16.4)	16.38 (2.94–24.53)	0
Boulad et al,[92] 2018	80	6	30.5 (21–34)	66.7	4	0	84.8 (65.6–89.9)	27.5 (7–132)[b]	NA	NA	1[d]
	160	3	32 (25–37)	33.3	2	1	74.9 (41.9–89.9)	43 (7–251)[b]	NA	NA	0
	240	6	34.5 (23–46)	83.3	4	0	79.6 (71.1–93.1)	30.5 (10–95)[b]	NA	NA	1[d]

Abbreviations: CD, cluster of differentiation; HU, hydroxyurea.
[a] Median (range).
[b] At 12 hours after plerixafor administration.
[c] Four severe VOCs and 1 delayed hemolytic transfusion reaction.
[d] Severe VOC.

leukocytapheresis products that may interfere with subsequent HSC purification and recovery.

SUMMARY

RBC and platelet transfusions are critical for treating SCD-associated complications and supporting patients during allogeneic and autologous HSCT. A major risk of transfusion therapy is RBC and HLA alloimmunization, for which contributing donor and recipient factors warrant consideration for HSCT donor selection and peri-HSCT transfusion support. HSCT is currently the only cure for SCD, but promising progress in novel gene therapy approaches may broaden accessibility to curative therapies in the near future.

DISCLOSURE

The authors have nothing to disclose.

REFERENCES

1. Vichinsky EP, Earles A, Johnson RA, et al. Alloimmunization in sickle cell anemia and transfusion of racially unmatched blood. N Engl J Med 1990;322(23): 1617–21.
2. Chou ST, Alsawas M, Fasano RM, et al. American Society of Hematology 2020 guidelines for sickle cell disease: transfusion support. Blood Adv 2020;4(2): 327–55.
3. Yawn BP, Buchanan GR, Afenyi-Annan AN, et al. Management of sickle cell disease: summary of the 2014 evidence-based report by expert panel members. JAMA 2014;312(10):1033–48.
4. Davis BA, Allard S, Qureshi A, et al. Guidelines on red cell transfusion in sickle cell disease Part II: indications for transfusion. Br J Haematol 2017;176(2): 192–209.
5. Stussi G, Buser A, Holbro A. Red blood cells: exchange, transfuse, or deplete. Transfus Med Hemother 2019;46(6):407–16.
6. Ware HM, Kwiatkowski JL. Evaluation and treatment of transfusional iron overload in children. Pediatr Clin North Am 2013;60(6):1393–406.
7. Biller E, Zhao Y, Berg M, et al. Red blood cell exchange in patients with sickle cell disease-indications and management: a review and consensus report by the therapeutic apheresis subsection of the AABB. Transfusion 2018;58(8): 1965–72.
8. Padmanabhan A, Connelly-Smith L, Aqui N, et al. Guidelines on the use of therapeutic apheresis in clinical practice - evidence-based approach from the Writing Committee of the American Society for apheresis: the Eighth special Issue. J Clin Apher 2019;34(3):171–354.
9. Venkateswaran L, Teruya J, Bustillos C, et al. Red cell exchange does not appear to increase the rate of allo- and auto-immunization in chronically transfused children with sickle cell disease. Pediatr Blood Cancer 2011;57(2):294–6.
10. Kassim AA, Galadanci NA, Pruthi S, et al. How I treat and manage strokes in sickle cell disease. Blood 2015;125(22):3401–10.
11. Adams RJ, McKie VC, Hsu L, et al. Prevention of a first stroke by transfusions in children with sickle cell anemia and abnormal results on transcranial Doppler ultrasonography. N Engl J Med 1998;339(1):5–11.

12. Lee MT, Piomelli S, Granger S, et al. Stroke prevention trial in sickle cell anemia (STOP): extended follow-up and final results. Blood 2006;108(3):847–52.

13. Adams RJ, Brambilla D. Discontinuing prophylactic transfusions used to prevent stroke in sickle cell disease. N Engl J Med 2005;353(26):2769–78.

14. Ware RE, Davis BR, Schultz WH, et al. Hydroxycarbamide versus chronic transfusion for maintenance of transcranial Doppler flow velocities in children with sickle cell anaemia-TCD with Transfusions Changing to Hydroxyurea (TWiTCH): a multicentre, open-label, phase 3, non-inferiority trial. Lancet 2016;387(10019): 661–70.

15. Powars D, Wilson B, Imbus C, et al. The natural history of stroke in sickle cell disease. Am J Med 1978;65(3):461–71.

16. Scothorn DJ, Price C, Schwartz D, et al. Risk of recurrent stroke in children with sickle cell disease receiving blood transfusion therapy for at least five years after initial stroke. J Pediatr 2002;140(3):348–54.

17. Hulbert ML, McKinstry RC, Lacey JL, et al. Silent cerebral infarcts occur despite regular blood transfusion therapy after first strokes in children with sickle cell disease. Blood 2011;117(3):772–9.

18. Ware RE, Helms RW. Stroke with transfusions changing to hydroxyurea (SWiTCH). Blood 2012;119(17):3925–32.

19. Kwiatkowski JL, Zimmerman RA, Pollock AN, et al. Silent infarcts in young children with sickle cell disease. Br J Haematol 2009;146(3):300–5.

20. Pegelow CH, Macklin EA, Moser FG, et al. Longitudinal changes in brain magnetic resonance imaging findings in children with sickle cell disease. Blood 2002;99(8):3014–8.

21. Schatz J, Brown RT, Pascual JM, et al. Poor school and cognitive functioning with silent cerebral infarcts and sickle cell disease. Neurology 2001;56(8): 1109–11.

22. Miller ST, Macklin EA, Pegelow CH, et al. Silent infarction as a risk factor for overt stroke in children with sickle cell anemia: a report from the Cooperative Study of Sickle Cell Disease. J Pediatr 2001;139(3):385–90.

23. DeBaun MR, Gordon M, McKinstry RC, et al. Controlled trial of transfusions for silent cerebral infarcts in sickle cell anemia. N Engl J Med 2014;371(8):699–710.

24. Platt OS, Brambilla DJ, Rosse WF, et al. Mortality in sickle cell disease. Life expectancy and risk factors for early death. N Engl J Med 1994;330(23):1639–44.

25. Vichinsky EP, Neumayr LD, Earles AN, et al. Causes and outcomes of the acute chest syndrome in sickle cell disease. National Acute Chest Syndrome Study Group. N Engl J Med 2000;342(25):1855–65.

26. Turner JM, Kaplan JB, Cohen HW, et al. Exchange versus simple transfusion for acute chest syndrome in sickle cell anemia adults. Transfusion 2009;49(5): 863–8.

27. Saylors RL, Watkins B, Saccente S, et al. Comparison of automated red cell exchange transfusion and simple transfusion for the treatment of children with sickle cell disease acute chest syndrome. Pediatr Blood Cancer 2013;60(12): 1952–6.

28. Emre U, Miller ST, Gutierez M, et al. Effect of transfusion in acute chest syndrome of sickle cell disease. J Pediatr 1995;127(6):901–4.

29. Castro O, Brambilla DJ, Thorington B, et al. The acute chest syndrome in sickle cell disease: incidence and risk factors. The Cooperative Study of Sickle Cell Disease. Blood 1994;84(2):643–9.

30. Hankins J, Jeng M, Harris S, et al. Chronic transfusion therapy for children with sickle cell disease and recurrent acute chest syndrome. J Pediatr Hematol Oncol 2005;27(3):158–61.

31. Howard J, Malfroy M, Llewelyn C, et al. The Transfusion Alternatives Preoperatively in Sickle Cell Disease (TAPS) study: a randomised, controlled, multicentre clinical trial. Lancet 2013;381(9870):930–8.

32. Vichinsky EP, Haberkern CM, Neumayr L, et al. A comparison of conservative and aggressive transfusion regimens in the perioperative management of sickle cell disease. The Preoperative Transfusion in Sickle Cell Disease Study Group. N Engl J Med 1995;333(4):206–13.

33. Nickel RS, Hendrickson JE, Fasano RM, et al. Impact of red blood cell alloimmunization on sickle cell disease mortality: a case series. Transfusion 2016;56(1):107–14.

34. Telen MJ, Afenyi-Annan A, Garrett ME, et al. Alloimmunization in sickle cell disease: changing antibody specificities and association with chronic pain and decreased survival. Transfusion 2015;55(6 Pt 2):1378–87.

35. Pirenne F, Yazdanbakhsh K. How I safely transfuse patients with sickle-cell disease and manage delayed hemolytic transfusion reactions. Blood 2018;131(25):2773–81.

36. Coleman S, Westhoff CM, Friedman DF, et al. Alloimmunization in patients with sickle cell disease and underrecognition of accompanying delayed hemolytic transfusion reactions. Transfusion 2019;59(7):2282–91.

37. Davis BA, Allard S, Qureshi A, et al. Guidelines on red cell transfusion in sickle cell disease. Part I: principles and laboratory aspects. Br J Haematol 2017;176(2):179–91.

38. Karafin MS, Westlake M, Hauser RG, et al. Risk factors for red blood cell alloimmunization in the Recipient Epidemiology and Donor Evaluation Study (REDS-III) database. Br J Haematol 2018;181(5):672–81.

39. Chou ST, Liem RI, Thompson AA. Challenges of alloimmunization in patients with haemoglobinopathies. Br J Haematol 2012;159(4):394–404.

40. Chou ST, Jackson T, Vege S, et al. High prevalence of red blood cell alloimmunization in sickle cell disease despite transfusion from Rh-matched minority donors. Blood 2013;122(6):1062–71.

41. Sakhalkar VS, Roberts K, Hawthorne LM, et al. Allosensitization in patients receiving multiple blood transfusions. Ann N Y Acad Sci 2005;1054:495–9.

42. Vichinsky EP, Luban NL, Wright E, et al. Prospective RBC phenotype matching in a stroke-prevention trial in sickle cell anemia: a multicenter transfusion trial. Transfusion 2001;41(9):1086–92.

43. Fasano RM, Booth GS, Miles M, et al. Red blood cell alloimmunization is influenced by recipient inflammatory state at time of transfusion in patients with sickle cell disease. Br J Haematol 2015;168(2):291–300.

44. Hudson KE, Fasano RM, Karafin MS, et al. Mechanisms of alloimmunization in sickle cell disease. Curr Opin Hematol 2019;26(6):434–41.

45. Casas J, Friedman DF, Jackson T, et al. Changing practice: red blood cell typing by molecular methods for patients with sickle cell disease. Transfusion 2015;55(6pt2):1388–93.

46. Lasalle-Williams M, Nuss R, Le T, et al. Extended red blood cell antigen matching for transfusions in sickle cell disease: a review of a 14-year experience from a single center (CME). Transfusion 2011;51(8):1732–9.

47. Chou ST, Fasano RM. Management of patients with sickle cell disease using transfusion therapy: guidelines and complications. Hematol Oncol Clin North Am 2016;30(3):591–608.

48. Fasano RM, Meyer EK, Branscomb J, et al. Impact of red blood cell antigen matching on alloimmunization and transfusion complications in patients with sickle cell disease: a systematic review. Transfus Med Rev 2019;33(1):12–23.

49. Tournamille C, Colin Y, Cartron JP, et al. Disruption of a GATA motif in the Duffy gene promoter abolishes erythroid gene expression in Duffy-negative individuals. Nat Genet 1995;10(2):224–8.

50. Kappler-Gratias S, Auxerre C, Dubeaux I, et al. Systematic RH genotyping and variant identification in French donors of African origin. Blood Transfus 2014; 12(Suppl 1):s264–72.

51. Gaspardi AC, Sippert EA, De Macedo MD, et al. Clinically relevant RHD-CE genotypes in patients with sickle cell disease and in African Brazilian donors. Blood Transfus 2016;14(5):449–54.

52. Wagner FF, Flegel WA. The Rhesus site. Transfus Med Hemother 2014;41(5): 357–63.

53. Blumenfeld OO, Patnaik SK. Allelic genes of blood group antigens: a source of human mutations and cSNPs documented in the Blood Group Antigen Gene Mutation Database. Hum Mutat 2004;23(1):8–16.

54. Chou ST, Evans P, Vege S, et al. RH genotype matching for transfusion support in sickle cell disease. Blood 2018;132(11):1198–207.

55. Marsella M, Borgna-Pignatti C. Transfusional iron overload and iron chelation therapy in thalassemia major and sickle cell disease. Hematol Oncol Clin North Am 2014;28(4):703–27, vi.

56. Meloni A, Puliyel M, Pepe A, et al. Cardiac iron overload in sickle-cell disease. Am J Hematol 2014;89(7):678–83.

57. de Montalembert M, Ribeil JA, Brousse V, et al. Cardiac iron overload in chronically transfused patients with thalassemia, sickle cell anemia, or myelodysplastic syndrome. PLoS One 2017;12(3):e0172147.

58. Kaushik N, Eckrich MJ, Parra D, et al. Chronically transfused pediatric sickle cell patients are protected from cardiac iron overload. Pediatr Hematol Oncol 2012; 29(3):254–60.

59. Brittenham GM, Cohen AR, McLaren CE, et al. Hepatic iron stores and plasma ferritin concentration in patients with sickle cell anemia and thalassemia major. Am J Hematol 1993;42(1):81–5.

60. Anwar M, Wood J, Manwani D, et al. Hepatic iron Quantification on 3 Tesla (3 T) magnetic resonance (MR): Technical challenges and Solutions. Radiol Res Pract 2013;2013:628150.

61. Angelucci E, Brittenham GM, McLaren CE, et al. Hepatic iron concentration and total body iron stores in thalassemia major. N Engl J Med 2000;343(5):327–31.

62. Wood JC, Enriquez C, Ghugre N, et al. MRI R2 and R2* mapping accurately estimates hepatic iron concentration in transfusion-dependent thalassemia and sickle cell disease patients. Blood 2005;106(4):1460–5.

63. St Pierre TG, Clark PR, Chua-anusorn W, et al. Noninvasive measurement and imaging of liver iron concentrations using proton magnetic resonance. Blood 2005;105(2):855–61.

64. Johnson FL, Look AT, Gockerman J, et al. Bone-marrow transplantation in a patient with sickle-cell anemia. N Engl J Med 1984;311(12):780–3.

65. Gluckman E, Cappelli B, Bernaudin F, et al. Sickle cell disease: an international survey of results of HLA-identical sibling hematopoietic stem cell transplantation. Blood 2017;129(11):1548–56.

66. Tanhehco YC, Bhatia M. Hematopoietic stem cell transplantation and cellular therapy in sickle cell disease: where are we now? Curr Opin Hematol 2019; 26(6):448–52.

67. Park SY, Matte A, Jung Y, et al. Pathologic angiogenesis in the bone marrow of humanized sickle cell mice is reversed by blood transfusion. Blood 2020; 135(23):2071–84.

68. Walters MC, Sullivan KM, Bernaudin F, et al. Neurologic complications after allogeneic marrow transplantation for sickle cell anemia. Blood 1995;85(4):879–84.

69. Cushing MM, Hendrickson JE. Transfusion support for hematopoietic stem cell transplant recipients. In: Fung MK, Anne E, Spitalnik SL, et al, editors. Technical manual. 19th edition. Bethesda, MD: AABB; 2017. p. 683–94.

70. Webb J, Abraham A. Complex transfusion issues in pediatric hematopoietic stem cell transplantation. Transfus Med Rev 2016;30(4):202–8.

71. Griffith LM, McCoy JP Jr, Bolan CD, et al. Persistence of recipient plasma cells and anti-donor isohaemagglutinins in patients with delayed donor erythropoiesis after major ABO incompatible non-myeloablative haematopoietic cell transplantation. Br J Haematol 2005;128(5):668–75.

72. Hendrickson J, Fasano R. Transfusion support of the patient with sickle cell disease undergoing transplantation. In:2018:111-136.

73. McPherson ME, Anderson AR, Haight AE, et al. Transfusion management of sickle cell patients during bone marrow transplantation with matched sibling donor. Transfusion 2009;49(9):1977–86.

74. Nickel RS, Flegel WA, Adams SD, et al. The impact of pre-existing HLA and red blood cell antibodies on transfusion support and engraftment in sickle cell disease after nonmyeloablative hematopoietic stem cell transplantation from HLA-matched sibling donors: a prospective, single-center, observational study. EClinicalMedicine 2020;24:100432.

75. Allen ES, Srivastava K, Hsieh MM, et al. Immunohaematological complications in patients with sickle cell disease after haemopoietic progenitor cell transplantation: a prospective, single-centre, observational study. Lancet Haematol 2017; 4(11):E553–61.

76. Nickel RS, Horan JT, Abraham A, et al. Human leukocyte antigen (HLA) class I antibodies and transfusion support in paediatric HLA-matched haematopoietic cell transplant for sickle cell disease. Br J Haematol 2020;189(1):162–70.

77. Vande Vusse LK, Madtes DK, Guthrie KA, et al. The association between red blood cell and platelet transfusion and subsequently developing idiopathic pneumonia syndrome after hematopoietic stem cell transplantation. Transfusion 2014;54(4):1071–80.

78. Solh M, Morgan S, McCullough J, et al. Blood transfusions and pulmonary complications after hematopoietic cell transplantation. Transfusion 2016;56(3): 653–61.

79. Gragert L, Eapen M, Williams E, et al. HLA match likelihoods for hematopoietic stem-cell grafts in the U.S. registry. N Engl J Med 2014;371(4):339–48.

80. Bolaños-Meade J, Fuchs EJ, Luznik L, et al. HLA-haploidentical bone marrow transplantation with posttransplant cyclophosphamide expands the donor pool for patients with sickle cell disease. Blood 2012;120(22):4285–91.

81. Dallas MH, Triplett B, Shook DR, et al. Long-term outcome and evaluation of organ function in pediatric patients undergoing haploidentical and matched

related hematopoietic cell transplantation for sickle cell disease. Biol Blood Marrow Transplant 2013;19(5):820–30.

82. Kamani NR, Walters MC, Carter S, et al. Unrelated donor cord blood transplantation for children with severe sickle cell disease: results of one cohort from the phase II study from the Blood and Marrow Transplant Clinical Trials Network (BMT CTN). Biol Blood Marrow Transplant 2012;18(8):1265–72.

83. Ruggeri A, Eapen M, Scaravadou A, et al. Umbilical cord blood transplantation for children with thalassemia and sickle cell disease. Biol Blood Marrow Transplant 2011;17(9):1375–82.

84. Esrick EB, Bauer DE. Genetic therapies for sickle cell disease. Semin Hematol 2018;55(2):76–86.

85. Tzounakas VL, Valsami SI, Kriebardis AG, et al. Red cell transfusion in paediatric patients with thalassaemia and sickle cell disease: current status, challenges and perspectives. Transfus Apher Sci 2018;57(3):347–57.

86. Ribeil J-A, Hacein-Bey-Abina S, Payen E, et al. Gene therapy in a patient with sickle cell disease. N Engl J Med 2017;376(9):848–55.

87. Adler BK, Salzman DE, Carabasi MH, et al. Fatal sickle cell crisis after granulocyte colony-stimulating factor administration. Blood 2001;97(10):3313–4.

88. Fitzhugh CD, Hsieh MM, Bolan CD, et al. Granulocyte colony-stimulating factor (G-CSF) administration in individuals with sickle cell disease: time for a moratorium? Cytotherapy 2009;11(4):464–71.

89. Abboud M, Laver J, Blau CA. Granulocytosis causing sickle-cell crisis. Lancet 1998;351(9107):959.

90. Esrick EB, Manis JP, Daley H, et al. Successful hematopoietic stem cell mobilization and apheresis collection using plerixafor alone in sickle cell patients. Blood Adv 2018;2(19):2505–12.

91. Lagresle-Peyrou C, Lefrère F, Magrin E, et al. Plerixafor enables safe, rapid, efficient mobilization of hematopoietic stem cells in sickle cell disease patients after exchange transfusion. Haematologica 2018;103(5):778–86.

92. Boulad F, Shore T, van Besien K, et al. Safety and efficacy of plerixafor dose escalation for the mobilization of CD34(+) hematopoietic progenitor cells in patients with sickle cell disease: interim results. Haematologica 2018;103(5): 770–7.

93. Uchida N, Leonard A, Stroncek D, et al. Safe and efficient peripheral blood stem cell collection in patients with sickle cell disease using plerixafor. Haematologica 2020. https://doi.org/10.3324/haematol.2019.236182.

94. Allen ES, Conry-Cantilena C. Mobilization and collection of cells in the hematologic compartment for cellular therapies: stem cell collection with G-CSF/plerixafor, collecting lymphocytes/monocytes. Semin Hematol 2019;56(4): 248–56.

95. Bujko K, Kucia M, Ratajczak J, et al. Hematopoietic stem and progenitor cells (HSPCs). In: Ratajczak MZ, editor. Stem cells: therapeutic applications. Cham (Switzerland): Springer International Publishing; 2019. p. 49–77.

96. Fukuda S, Bian H, King AG, et al. The chemokine GRObeta mobilizes early hematopoietic stem cells characterized by enhanced homing and engraftment. Blood 2007;110(3):860–9.

97. Hoggatt J, Singh P, Tate TA, et al. Rapid mobilization reveals a highly engraftable hematopoietic stem cell. Cell 2018;172(1–2):191–204.e10.

98. Richard RE, Siritanaratkul N, Jonlin E, et al. Collection of blood stem cells from patients with sickle cell anemia. Blood Cells Mol Dis 2005;35(3):384–8.

99. Yannaki E, Papayannopoulou T, Jonlin E, et al. Hematopoietic stem cell mobilization for gene therapy of adult patients with severe β-thalassemia: results of clinical trials using G-CSF or plerixafor in splenectomized and nonsplenectomized subjects. Mol Ther 2012;20(1):230–8.
100. Constantinou VC, Bouinta A, Karponi G, et al. Poor stem cell harvest may not always be related to poor mobilization: lessons gained from a mobilization study in patients with β-thalassemia major. Transfusion 2017;57(4):1031–9.

Cellular Therapy in Pediatric Hematologic Malignancies

Susan Kuldanek, MD[a], Bryce Pasko, MD[b,d], Melkon DomBourian, MD[c,d],
Kyle Annen, DO[b,d,*]

KEYWORDS

- CAR T cell • HPSC • Pediatric • Regulatory • NK cell therapy
- Cord blood expansion

KEY POINTS

- Hematopoietic stem cell (HPSC) transplant is the most common and standardized cellular therapy. Advances such as using haploidentical matches have improved the available donor pool, and product manipulations such as αβ T-cell depletion show an improved safety profile and reduced risk of complications such as graft-versus-host disease and infection caused by delayed engraftment.
- Chimeric antigen receptor therapies have provided an essential bridge to HPSC transplant for patients with relapsed/refractory leukemia and may prove to be an effective stand-alone therapy.
- Regulatory T cells show promise as an alternative to common medications with a high side effect profile, such as glucocorticoids.
- Natural killer cells are a focus of current studies, both for enhancement within HPSC grafts and for stand-alone therapy. Their unique profile as a part of the innate immune system makes them an ideal target for future treatments.
- The Foundation for the Accreditation of Cellular Therapies in collaboration with the international Joint Accreditation Committee provides guidance on maintaining the safety, purity, and potency of cellular therapies.

[a] Hemophilia and Thrombosis Center, Center for Cancer and Blood Disorders, Children's Hospital Colorado, University of Colorado-Anschutz Medical Campus, 13123 East 16th Avenue, Aurora, CO 80045, USA; [b] Department of Pathology and Laboratory Medicine, University of Colorado-Anschutz Medical Campus, Aurora, CO, USA; [c] Main Core Laboratory and Point of Care Testing, Department of Pathology and Laboratory Medicine, Children's Hospital Colorado, 13123 East 16th Avenue, B120, Aurora, CO 80045, USA; [d] Department of Pathology, University of Colorado-Anschutz Medical Campus, Aurora, CO, USA
* Corresponding author. Department of Pathology and Laboratory Medicine, Children's Hospital Colorado, 13123 East 16th Avenue, B120, Aurora, CO 80045.
E-mail address: kyle.annen@childrenscolorado.org

Clin Lab Med 41 (2021) 121–132
https://doi.org/10.1016/j.cll.2020.10.008 labmed.theclinics.com
0272-2712/21/© 2020 Elsevier Inc. All rights reserved.

INTRODUCTION

Cellular therapy for pediatric hematologic malignancies has made significant advances in recent years. New technologies for hematopoietic stem cell transplant allow broadened opportunities for finding a suitable donor (eg, haploidentical), as well as manipulations such as αß T-cell depletions and umbilical cord blood expansion. The development of Chimeric antigen receptor (CAR) T-cell therapy has resulted in a significant improvement in mortality for relapsed/refractory leukemia. CAR technology shows promise as other cell lines are developed into adoptive therapies, including natural killer cells and regulatory T cells (Tregs). Regulatory requirements must keep up with these advances, which sometimes causes confusion. These topics are highlighted and addressed in this article.

HEMATOPOIETIC STEM CELL TRANSPLANT

Hematopoietic stem cell transplant (HSCT) is the first cellular therapy used in patients with hematopoietic malignancies for curative intent. The earliest example of its use dates back to 1959 when 2 patients, each with an identical twin, with advanced acute lymphoblastic leukemia (ALL) were infused with syngeneic marrow following a conditioning regimen of lethal total body irradiation (TBI). Both patients engrafted within weeks, but ultimately died of relapsed disease.[1]

Allogeneic grafts are used in pediatric hematologic malignancies, given both the concern for malignant contamination with autologous infusion as well as the added beneficial graft-versus-leukemia effect seen with allogeneic graft infusion. Recognition of major histocompatibility complex (MHC) molecules by T cells, known as alloimmunity, is the basis for graft rejection and graft-versus-host disease (GVHD). Graft rejection, defined as the failure to recover hematopoietic function by day +100, is affected not only by human leukocyte antigen (HLA) mismatch but also by graft source, lower hematopoietic stem cell (HSC) dose, T-cell depletion, and a history of multiple transfusions. Histocompatibility testing generally includes the MHC class I molecules HLA-A, HLA-B, and HLA-C, and the MHC class II molecules HLA-DR, HLA-DQ, and HLA-DP. These markers are inherited as a haplotype; hence, every full sibling confers a 25% chance of being a perfect match with the additional advantage of matching for minor histocompatibility antigens, thus decreasing risk for nonengraftment and GVHD. However, only about 30% of patients have an HLA-matched sibling. With continued improvements in GVHD prevention, alternative graft sources have increased the availability of appropriately matched donors, particularly for patients of nonwhite ethnic makeup. Alternative donors include mismatched related donor, matched unrelated donor, umbilical cord blood (UCB), and, more recently, haploidentical hematopoietic stem cells. Bone marrow is primarily used as the HSC source in pediatrics rather than peripherally (apheresis) derived collections because of the higher risks of chronic GVHD, treatment-related mortality (TRM), and overall mortality associated with the use of peripherally derived HSCs.[2] This approach is in contrast with adult patients, in whom peripherally derived HSCs are favored because of improved mortality and TRM. T-cell depletion ex vivo reduces the risk of GVHD and, in the setting of haploidentical transplant, has allowed transplant in the approximately 60% to 70% of children lacking a fully matched donor while relying on the innate antileukemic functioning of natural killer (NK) cells.[3–5] Historically, haploidentical transplant was associated with high morbidity and mortality resulting from relapse, GVHD, and infection caused by delayed immune reconstitution. However, newer technologies that allow high-purity cluster of differentiation (CD) 34+ cell selection, while excluding alloreactive T and B cells, have mitigated these complications to some degree. Each methodology has its own set of advantages and disadvantages.[4] Expanded cord technologies for patients without a suitable HLA-matched donor are under current investigation in both clinical trials and murine models.[6]

Engraftment kinetics vary by graft source, HSC number, preinfusion manipulations, as well as GVHD prophylaxis. Engraftment is generally enhanced by the use of growth factors, most commonly granulocyte colony-stimulating factor (GCSF). Neutrophil recovery occurs first generally about 2 to 3 weeks from the bone marrow-derived HSC infusion (denoted as day 0) and is followed by platelet recovery 1 to 2 weeks later.[7] Kinetics are increased by 1 to 7 days when peripherally derived HSCs are used and delayed with the use of UCB HSCs.[8] Bacterial and fungal infections are important causes of TRM before myeloid engraftment, and delayed engraftment strongly affects infectious risks. Patients remain susceptible to viral infections for at least 1 year after HSCT because of cellular immune dysfunction despite normal numbers of circulating lymphocytes. T-cell reductive therapies further increase viral susceptibility, of which cytomegalovirus (CMV) is a particular concern, and antiviral medications decrease overall mortality. Treatment with steroids for GVHD or other complications further increases patient susceptibility, particularly to fungal infection. Prophylaxis to prevent *Pneumocystis jiroveci* following transplant is standard.

Multiple factors, most importantly, the degree of HLA matching but also the use of TBI, are important risk factors for GVHD. GVHD, both acute and chronic, are important mediators of morbidity and mortality. Damage to the skin, liver, and lower gastrointestinal system arises from direct killing of host cells by alloantigen-specific T cells and by damage induced by inflammatory mediators. Umbilical cord blood transplant confers the lowest risk for GVHD, although infectious complications remain high given the slower engraftment rates as well as the relative immunologic naivety of the graft.[9] Other noninfectious complications arise from toxicities associated with the conditioning regimen, infection from myelosuppression, and immune-mediated reactions. Conditioning, generally chemotherapy and/or radiotherapy, serves several purposes, including creating space in the marrow niche, providing appropriate immunosuppression to allow HSC engraftment, and targeting and destroying any residual malignant cells. Preexisting iron overload and active infection at the time of transplant further increase the risk of complications.[10] Several distinct syndromes arise as the result of endothelial damage induced by proinflammatory, prothrombotic, and proapoptotic changes related to the conditioning regimen, the administration of GCSF and/or immunomodulatory agents, and the onset of leukocyte engraftment.[11] Sinusoidal obstruction syndrome/veno-occlusive disease (VOD) is a potentially life-threatening condition caused by damage to the sinusoidal endothelial cells and hepatocytes by exposure to toxic metabolites during conditioning, particularly those associated with myeloablative regimens. Endothelial cell activation and damage, platelet adhesion, local immune reactivity, cellular egress, venule narrowing, and reduced sinusoidal blood flow result in the clinical constellation of tender hepatomegaly, weight gain from ascites, and hyperbilirubinemia.[12] Inflammatory syndromes may occur and include engraftment syndrome, characterized by massive cytokine release; capillary leak syndrome, involving interstitial fluid accumulation; and diffuse alveolar hemorrhage, which involves red blood cell extravasation into the alveoli. Transplant-associated thrombocytopenic microangiopathy, associated with thrombocytopenia, evidence of hemolysis (schistocytes on smear, increased lactate dehydrogenase and bilirubin levels, and decreased haptoglobin), and organ failure often occurs in the first 20 to 60 days following transplant and is associated with high morbidity rates. Conditioning agents, as well as calcineurin inhibitors, seem to play a role in inducing endothelial damage and platelet microthrombi formation. Plasma exchange tends not to be helpful, but terminal complement inhibitors such as eculizumab play a role in treating this process.[13] Basic science work corroborates clinical observations that inflammatory phenotypes, such as engraftment syndrome and capillary leak syndrome, occur with greater frequency in autologous transplant versus conditions with a prothrombotic phenotype, such as transplant-associated microangiopathy and VOD, which predominate in allogeneic transplant.[11] Long-term complications are many and beyond the scope of this article, but may involve all the major organ systems and lead to long-term growth and neurologic problems, cytopenias, and secondary malignancy.

CHIMERIC ANTIGEN RECEPTOR T-CELL THERAPY

Most patients who fail standard chemotherapy regimens are either refractory to therapy or relapse following transplant: approximately 3%, and up to 15%, respectively.[14] Immunotherapy, in particular CAR T-cell therapy, has revolutionized refractory/relapsed (R/R) patient management, with 1-year clinical remission in up to 90% of R/R patients treated with CAR T-cell therapy.[15]

Current CAR T-cell therapy uses autologous T cells collected via peripheral blood mononuclear cell collection. These T cells, predominantly CD3+, are then reprogramed using a retrovirus or lentivirus vector to insert a binding domain that allows the new transduced T cells to target tumor cell surface markers, such as CD19+ cells in ALL. The CAR constructs have a modified intracellular domain, transmembrane domain, hinge region, and costimulatory domain. These modifications allow the T cells to work similarly to an antibody that targets and binds specific cell surface markers, leading to the destruction of all cells with the targeted surface marker. Once modified, the CAR constructs are expanded to a concentration that is sufficient to infuse into the patient and have a potent antitumor effect.[16–18] Once reinfused, the CAR T constructs target and destroy all cells with the CAR program targeted surface marker; for example, CD19-positive B cells in B-cell ALL (B-ALL). CARs also have on-target, but off-site, cell destruction, which can lead to a complete B-cell aplasia.[19]

The major side effects of CAR T-cell therapy are cytokine release syndrome (CRS) and immune effector cell–associated neurotoxicity syndrome (ICANS). CRS and the early-phase component of ICANS are associated with the rapid destruction of the targeted cells. For this reason, many patients are treated with chemotherapy before infusion of the CAR T-cell product, to minimize the disease burden and the risk of severe CRS and early-phase ICANS, while improving the efficacy of the CAR T product.[18,20,21] Tocilizumab, a monoclonal antibody against interleukin (IL)-6 receptors, is effective in treating the CRS and early-phase ICANS without adversely affecting the efficacy of the CAR T-cell therapy.[21–23]

In 2017, the US Food and Drug Administration (FDA) approved 2 separate CAR T-cell therapies following their tremendous success in randomized controlled trials. Tisagenlecleucel (Kymriah, Novartis) for the treatment of R/R patients less than 25 years old with B-ALL, then later for non-Hodgkin lymphoma, and axicabtagene ciloleucel (Yescarta, KITE/Gilead), for the treatment of diffuse large B-cell lymphoma.[24–26] In pediatric patients with R/R B-ALL, tisagenlecleucel is used predominantly as a bridge to bone marrow transplant.[24] With the significant successes of CAR T-cell therapy, research is expanding around the globe. As of August 5, 2020, there are 662 active ongoing CAR T trials in the United States, of which 235 are for children between birth and 17 years old when searching clinicaltrials.gov using the criteria: not yet recruiting, recruiting, enrolling by invitation, or active not recruiting.

Future directions for CAR T-cell therapy include increasing the number of indications and CAR targets, improving the manufacturing process, and expanding collections to include healthy allogeneic T-cell donors. As applications for CAR T therapies expand, it is essential to minimize the on-target, off-site effects, which is why current therapies have focused on tumor-isolated markers, such as solid tumors such as glioblastoma multiforme (IL-13), common pediatric brain tumors, and breast cancer (HER2), which have surface markers not found on most healthy tissues.[27] To increase manufacturing efficiency while reducing the massive demand for resources, manufacturers are working on creating automated closed systems for CAR manufacturing, such as the CliniMACS Prodigy & Cocoon.[16] In addition, having healthy allogeneic donors collected for modified or universal CAR T-cell therapy would markedly increase the availability of CARs for patients who are unable to produce their own T cells and would increase the availability of off-the-shelf targeted immunotherapies. Given the rapid changes to immunotherapy in the last 10 years, the future direction of CAR T-cell therapy is promising.

REGULATORY T CELLS

Tregs function to maintain self-immune tolerance and regulate the suppression of excessive immune responses.[28] Although postulated for some time, it was not until the mid-1990s that Tregs were shown to play a vital role in immune regulation.[29] They are characterized by an immunophenotype of $CD4^+CD25^{high}CD127^{low/-}FoxP3^+$ and work by inhibiting antigen-presenting cells, NK cells, B cells, and other T cells.[30] Successful preclinical animal studies have led to clinical trial work in various areas, including HSCT.[30]

One key to the therapeutic promise of Tregs is their targeted immunosuppressive properties being similar to traditional glucocorticoids but without the associated systemic side effects.[30,31] Their use in HSCT has generally been focused on the prevention of GVHD, and compassionate use in unresponsive patients has shown some efficacy in both acute and chronic forms of the disease.[32–34] Tregs can be collected from allogeneic or autologous sources and can be administered fresh or expanded as polyclonal or antigen-specific cell preparations.[30]

Treg levels are increased in several human cancers, including ALL, and it is postulated that Treg suppressive properties on cytotoxic cells could play a role in the faster spread of tumor cells.[35–37] Although pediatric studies are limited, those focused on ALL have shown that a higher percentage of Treg cells is seen in the peripheral blood and bone marrow of pediatric patients with ALL compared with healthy controls.[38] This increase of Treg level has been correlated with disease progression and is involved in downregulation NK cell function, and these findings suggest that Tregs may play a role in pediatric leukemia occurrence and development.[38,39] Further studies are needed for extrapolation to the general population of pediatric patients with ALL. However, these early studies suggest the possibility that routine determination of Treg characteristics in children with ALL could be used in the assessment of disease severity and prognosis and could potentially provide future therapeutic targets.

NATURAL KILLER CELL ADOPTIVE THERAPY

The success of CAR T cells in the treatment of leukemia and lymphoma has created an interest in exploring the development of other immune cell therapies. NK cells are lymphoid cells that lack surface T-cell receptors (CD3) and express neural cell adhesion molecules (CD56).[40] They are part of the innate immune system, and as such do not require prior exposure to an antigen. NK cells are $CD3^-$, $CD56^+/CD16^+$, and, when mature (CD56[dim]/CD16[bright]), they are highly cytotoxic. NK cells are "serial killers," in that the release of only a few granules may be enough to kill a target cell, and, once the cell is destroyed, the NK cells are able to attack additional targets.[41] Despite not requiring memory for the cytotoxic response, NK cells have been found to develop a memorylike function that enhances their targeting, which has been demonstrated against CMV, and also to develop a highly cytotoxic affinity to B-cell lineage leukemia with the expression of anti-CD19 signaling receptors.[42,43]

NK cells are enabled by a group of activating, costimulatory, and inhibitory receptors, of which the best known are NK-cell immunoglobulinlike receptors (KIRs), which are germline-encoded inhibitory receptors. NK-cell activation occurs when there is a loss of a cellular inhibitory signal caused by cancer or viral infection. When the inhibitor ligands (MHC class I) are no longer present, the KIR identifies the cell as nonself and attacks.[44,45] For HSCT, this results in an interesting relationship for the KIR nonself identification and destruction of cells, because KIR genes and HLA genes segregate independently, with only 25% of HLA-matched siblings also matched for KIR.[46] Early studies on KIR-mismatched HSCT for patients with acute myeloid leukemia (AML) found a significantly lower risk of relapse and improved overall survival; however, posttransplant cyclophosphamide, which is now routine, rapidly eliminates the early proliferation of NK cells, eliminating the benefit of NK KIR mismatch. Mismatched HSCT for pediatric solid tumors has shown a beneficial allograft-versus-tumor effect with early NK immune reconstitution.[47] In pediatric ALL, it has been documented that patients have a decreased cytotoxic NK-cell response, with an increased expression of inhibitory markers. The ability to supplement or augment NK cells may be useful as a therapeutic modality to improve outcomes.[48] NK cells are the first lymphocytes to reconstitute after HSCT and play a critical role in the graft-versus-tumor response. Further, NK cells may protect against GVHD by suppressing alloreactive T-cell responses.[49]

NK cells have been explored as a stand-alone therapy in the nontransplant setting with success in small clinical studies for patients with AML.[50,51] Clinical trials for autologous NK-cell therapy consist of autologous mononuclear cell apheresis collection, in vitro amplification for NK cells, and subsequent reinfusion.[51] Allogeneic NK infusions are also being studied; however, the KIR and HLA mismatch can be more challenging to manage.[52] This difficulty has led to increased interest in engineered NK cells; however, this may be a double-edged sword, in that, by not requiring a specific antigen for targeting, there is a disadvantage when engineering these cells for a specific cancer target. A significant potential advantage of NK therapy is that its development could be off the shelf: with a lack of T-cell surface receptors and no risk of GVHD, this therapy could be manufactured in advance and given to multiple patients, rather than the individualized process needed for CAR T-cell therapy.[40,52] CAR engineering is being used to develop NK cells for therapy in multiple preclinical studies, and a clinical trial testing the efficacy and safety of an off-the-shelf cord blood–derived NK product for refractory lymphoid malignancies is underway (NCT03056339). The NK cells engineering process is working to improve in vivo persistence, decreasing cytotoxicity, homing to the target cells, and eluding the immunosuppressive tumor microenvironment. Non–patient-specific therapies in development include bispecific killer engagers (BiKEs) and trispecific killer engagers (TriKEs). These therapies are small molecules containing a single variable portion of an antibody, which is linked to 1 (BiKE) or 2 (TriKEs) variable portions of other antibodies with a different specificity. By binding these to NK cells and targeting a specific tumor antigen, NK cells can be targeted to the desired cell.[53]

αβ AND T-CELL DEPLETIONS

Partial HLA-matched or haploidentical transplants have emerged as an option for transplant in light of the continued challenges in finding fully HLA-matched donors. Early haploidentical or partial HLA-matched HSCT results in high rates of graft failure, GVHD, and relapse. Haploidentical transplants also have long engraftment times, increasing morbidity and mortality because of infection and delayed immune reconstitution.[54] T-cell depletion was developed in the 1980s as an effective method of reducing GVHD and allowed decreased posttransplant immunosuppression, but at the cost of the antitumor and antiinfectious properties of the graft.[55–58] In response, an advanced method of depleting only T lymphocytes while retaining γδ+ T lymphocytes, NK cells, and other cells in the graft has been developed. This process simplifies a prior 2-step process into a single step by using magnetic microbeads coated with an αβ antibody, then passing the microbeads through a magnetic separation column, followed by elution of the targeted cells (CliniMACS, Miltenyi).[59,60] αβ+ depleted grafts have been shown to provide the benefits of T-cell depletion, particularly reduction in GVHD, while allowing the remaining γδ+ T cells to provide the antitumor and antiinfectious benefits, as well as more rapid reconstitution than CD3/CD19-depleted grafts.[54,59]

Studies in children with leukemia and lymphoma have shown promising results and further highlight the critical differences in the variable T-cell lines in immune reconstitution. One study in children with acute leukemia reported a reduced incidence of bacterial and fungal infections and higher levels of event-free survival in the first year following HSCT.[61,62] Other murine models highlight improvements in the gut microbiome, which may reduce opportunistic infection.[63] Improved ability to select for the desired immune cells for earlier engraftment, prevention of infection, and immune reconstitution has resulted in better outcomes and improved quality of life by reducing the incidence of GVHD and decreasing the severity of immunosuppressive chemotherapy.

REGULATORY CONSIDERATIONS IN THE UNITED STATES

The FDA Center for Biologics Evaluation and Research regulates cellular therapy products in the United States, including autologous and allogeneic collected cells as well as the cellular-based immunotherapies discussed earlier.[64] In addition to following FDA regulations and guidance, facilities can also seek voluntary cellular therapy–related accreditation through the Foundation for the Accreditation of Cellular Therapy (FACT) in collaboration with the international Joint Accreditation Committee (JACIE).[65] FACT-JACIE is sponsored jointly by the American Society for Transplantation and Cellular Therapy as well as the International Society for Cell & Gene Therapy and provides evidence-based standards for cellular therapy programs. Four primary standards have been developed: international standards for hematopoietic cellular therapy product collection, processing, and administration; immune effector cells; cord blood collection, banking and release for administration; and common standards for cellular therapies.[66] Within the common and hematopoietic and immune effector cell standards is pediatric-specific guidance for attending physicians' qualifications and education activities, procedural policies, and a minimum number of patients for accreditation.[67,68]

Facilities seeking FACT-JACIE accreditation for a single pediatric site need to have and maintain a minimum of 5 autologous or 10 allogeneic recipients over the prior 12 months. If a facility serves a combined adult and pediatric transplant population at a single site, it must have and maintain a minimum of 5 adult and 5 pediatric recipients for allogeneic and/or autologous transplants. There are additional requirements if the program serves multiple clinical sites.[66] Pediatric expertise is expected, with at least 1 attending physician required to have achieved certification in pediatric hematology/oncology or pediatric immunology, and all program faculty must complete a minimum of 10 hours annually of educational activities on cellular therapy with some related to HSCT.[67–69] Nursing staff and transplant teams must be trained in the management of pediatric donors and recipients. There should also be policies and procedures that address pediatric-specific considerations such as the impact on postcellular therapy, late effects on growth and development, and acceptance of pediatric recipients into long-term follow-up clinics as adults.[67]

Evidence of compliance for FACT-JACIE standards follows general laboratory medicine practice with documentation and reports. Specific guidance on how to meet the standards can be found in standard associated accreditation manuals.[65] Ultimately, the clinical program director or designee is the physician responsible for all elements of the cellular therapy program, including quality management systems, operating procedures, staff training, and clinical outcome analysis. The director or designee must also show regular interaction among clinical sites, as applicable.[68]

SUMMARY

HSCT has become the cornerstone of treatment of adult and pediatric patients with lymphoblastic T-cell and B-cell leukemias and lymphomas. Most pediatric cancers are treated with some combination of chemotherapy, radiation, surgical resection, immunotherapy, or HSCT. Pediatric cancer treatments and survival have improved significantly over the last 40 to 50 years. Methodologies and conditioning regimens have evolved dramatically over time and have resulted in improved mortality as well as quality of life during the transplant period. Modifications such as T-cell reduction and $\alpha\beta$ T-cell reduction have further optimized the transplant cell product. Newer treatment options such as CAR T-cell therapy are increasingly used to achieve pre-HSCT remission and, in some circumstances, as salvage therapy in patients with high-risk disease. Further refinements to conditioning regimens, graft manipulations, and alternative graft sources will continue to improve survival in patients with high-risk hematologic malignancies.

Adoptive cell therapy, such as the successful CAR T-cell therapies for relapsed/refractory pediatric leukemias, have provided a critical bridge to transplant and may prove to be effective as a stand-alone therapy. Additional CAR T-cell therapies are in development. NK cells are now understood to play an important role in the prevention of GVHD and immune reconstitution, as well as the graft-versus-leukemia response. Development of stand-alone therapies that could act like a CAR but do not need to be tailored to individual patients could provide a therapy that is more rapidly available than patient-specific CAR T treatments in their current form. Regulatory T cells show promise as a replacement for glucocorticoids and their accompanying side effects. All of these modalities are guided by the criteria set out by regulatory and accreditation bodies such as the FDA and FACT-JACIE, whose goals are to bring new treatment options to patients and to maintain high quality and safety for patients undergoing cellular therapies.

DISCLOSURE

K. Annen: consulting contract with Terumo BCT. The other authors have nothing to disclose.

REFERENCES

1. Thomas ED, Lochte HL Jr, Cannon JH, et al. Supralethal whole body irradiation and isologous marrow transplantation in man. J Clin Invest 1959;38:1709–16.
2. Eapen M, Horowitz MM, Klein JP, et al. Higher mortality after allogeneic peripheral-blood transplantation compared with bone marrow in children and adolescents: the histocompatibility and alternate stem cell source working Committee of the international bone marrow transplant Registry. J Clin Oncol 2004;22: 4872–80.
3. Cairo MS, Rocha V, Gluckman E, et al. Alternative allogeneic donor sources for transplantation for childhood diseases: unrelated cord blood and haploidentical family donors. Biol Blood Marrow Transplant 2008;14:44–53.
4. Gonzalez-Vicent M, Diaz Perez MA. Allogeneic hematopoietic stem-cell transplantation from haploidentical donors using 'ex-vivo' T-cell depletion in pediatric patients with hematological malignancies: state of the art review. Curr Opin Oncol 2018;30:396–401.
5. Ruggeri L, Capanni M, Urbani E, et al. Effectiveness of donor natural killer cell alloreactivity in mismatched hematopoietic transplants. Science 2002;295: 2097–100.
6. Cohen S, Roy J, Lachance S, et al. Hematopoietic stem cell transplantation using single UM171-expanded cord blood: a single-arm, phase 1-2 safety and feasibility study. Lancet Haematol 2020;7:e134–45.
7. Cutler C, Antin JH. Peripheral blood stem cells for allogeneic transplantation: a review. Stem Cells 2001;19:108–17.
8. Rocha V, Wagner JE Jr, Sobocinski KA, et al. Graft-versus-host disease in children who have received a cord-blood or bone marrow transplant from an HLA-identical sibling. Eurocord and international bone marrow transplant Registry working Committee on alternative donor and stem cell sources. N Engl J Med 2000;342:1846–54.
9. Gluckman E, Rocha V, Boyer-Chammard A, et al. Eurocord transplant group and the European blood and marrow transplantation GroupOutcome of cord-blood transplantation from related and unrelated donors. N Engl J Med 1997;337: 373–81.
10. Deeg HJ, Spaulding E, Shulman HM. Iron overload, hematopoietic cell transplantation, and graft-versus-host disease. Leuk Lymphoma 2009;50:1566–72.
11. Carreras E, Diaz-Ricart M. The role of the endothelium in the short-term complications of hematopoietic SCT. Transplant 2011;46:1495–502.
12. Mohty M, Malard F, Abecassis M, et al. Sinusoidal obstruction syndrome/veno-occlusive disease: current situation and perspectives-a position statement from the European Society for Blood and Marrow Transplantation (EBMT). Bone Marrow Transplant 2015;50:781–9.
13. Obut F, Kasinath V, Abdi R. Post-bone marrow transplant thrombotic microangiopathy. Bone Marrow Transplant 2016;51:891–7.
14. Schrappe M, Hunger SP, Pui CH, et al. Outcomes after induction failure in childhood acute lymphoblastic leukemia. N Engl J Med 2012;366:1371–81.
15. Hucks G, Rheingold SR. The journey to CAR T cell therapy: the pediatric and young adult experience with relapsed or refractory B-ALL. Blood Cancer J 2019;9(2):10.
16. Reddy OL, Stroncek DF, Panch SR. Improving CAR T cell therapy by optimizing critical quality attributes. Semin Hematol 2020;57(2):33–8.

17. Marple AH, Bonifant C, Shah NN. Improving CAR T-cells: the next generation. Semin Hematol 2020. https://doi.org/10.1053/j.seminhematol.2020.07.002.
18. Szenes V, Curran KJ. Utilization of CAR T cell therapy in pediatric patients. Semin Oncol Nurs 2019;35(5):150929.
19. Kansagra AJ, Frey NV, Bar M, et al. Clinical utilization of Chimeric antigen receptor T cells in B cell acute lymphoblastic leukemia: an expert Opinion from the European Society for blood and marrow transplantation and the American Society for blood and marrow transplantation. Biol Blood Marrow Transplant 2019; 25(3):e76–85.
20. Davila ML, Sadelain M. Biology and clinical application of CAR T cells for B cell malignancies. Int J Hematol 2016;104(1):6–17.
21. Lee DW, Santomasso BD, Locke FL, et al. ASTCT consensus grading for cytokine release syndrome and neurologic toxicity associated with immune effector cells. Biol Blood Marrow Transplant 2019;25(4):625–38.
22. Maude SL, Barrett D, Teachey DT, et al. Managing cytokine release syndrome associated with novel T cell-engaging therapies. Cancer J 2014;20(2):119–22.
23. Nishimoto N, Terao K, Mima T, et al. Mechanisms and pathologic significances in increase in serum interleukin-6 (IL-6) and soluble IL-6 receptor after administration of an anti-IL-6 receptor antibody, tocilizumab, in patients with rheumatoid arthritis and Castleman disease. Blood 2008;112(10):3959–64.
24. Maude SL, Laetsch TW, Buechner J, et al. Tisagenlecleucel in children and young adults with B-cell lymphoblastic leukemia. N Engl J Med 2018;378(5):439–48.
25. Schuster SJ, Bishop MR, Tam CS, et al. Tisagenlecleucel in adult relapsed or refractory diffuse large B-cell lymphoma. N Engl J Med 2019;380(1):45–56.
26. Locke FL, Ghobadi A, Jacobson CA, et al. Long-term safety and activity of axicabtagene ciloleucel in refractory large B-cell lymphoma (ZUMA-1): a single-arm, multicentre, phase 1–2 trial. Lancet Oncol 2019;20(1):31–42.
27. Subklewe M, von Bergwelt-Baildon M, Humpe A. Chimeric antigen receptor T cells: a race to revolutionize cancer therapy. Transfus Med Hemother 2019; 46(1):15–24.
28. Miyara M, Gorochov G, Ehrenstein M, et al. Human FoxP3+ regulatory T cells in systemic autoimmune diseases. Autoimmun Rev 2011;10(12):744–55.
29. Sakaguchi S, Sakaguchi N, Asano M, et al. Immunologic self-tolerance maintained by activated T cells expressing IL-2 receptor alpha-chains (CD25). Breakdown of a single mechanism of self-tolerance causes various autoimmune diseases. J Immunol 1995;155(3):1151–64.
30. Gliwiński M, Iwaszkiewicz-Grześ D, Trzonkowski P. Cell-Based Therapies with T regulatory cells. BioDrugs 2017;31(4):335–47.
31. Niedźwiecki M, Budziło O, Adamkiewicz-Drożyńska E, et al. CD4+CD25highCD127low/-FoxP3+ regulatory T-cell population in acute leukemias: a review of the literature. J Immunol Res 2019;2019:2816498.
32. Trzonkowski P, Bieniaszewska M, Juścińska J, et al. First-in-man clinical results of the treatment of patients with graft versus host disease with human ex vivo expanded CD4+CD25+CD127- T regulatory cells. Clin Immunol 2009; 133(1):22–6.
33. Brunstein CG, Miller JS, Cao Q, et al. Infusion of ex vivo expanded T regulatory cells in adults transplanted with umbilical cord blood: safety profile and detection kinetics. Blood 2011;117(3):1061–70.
34. Brunstein CG, Miller JS, McKenna DH, et al. Umbilical cord blood-derived T regulatory cells to prevent GVHD: kinetics, toxicity profile, and clinical effect. Blood 2016;127(8):1044–51.

35. Niedźwiecki M, Budziło O, Zieliński M, et al. CD4+CD25highCD127low/-FoxP3+ regulatory T cell Subpopulations in the bone marrow and peripheral blood of children with ALL: brief Report. J Immunol Res 2018;2018:1292404.

36. Trzonkowski P, Szmit E, Myśliwska J, et al. CD4+CD25+ T regulatory cells inhibit cytotoxic activity of T CD8+ and NK lymphocytes in the direct cell-to-cell interaction. Clin Immunol 2004;112(3):258–67.

37. Li Q, Egilmez NK. Ontogeny of tumor-associated CD4+CD25+Foxp3+ T-regulatory cells. Immunol Invest 2016;45(8):729–45.

38. Bhattacharya K, Chandra S, Mandal C. Critical stoichiometric ratio of CD4(+) CD25(+) FoxP3(+) regulatory T cells and CD4(+) CD25(-) responder T cells influence immunosuppression in patients with B-cell acute lymphoblastic leukaemia. Immunology 2014;142(1):124–39.

39. Wu ZL, Hu GY, Chen FX, et al. Change of CD4(+) CD25(+) regulatory T cells and NK Cells in peripheral blood of children with acute leukemia and its possible significance in tumor immunity. Zhongguo Shi Yan Xue Ye Xue Za Zhi 2010;18(3):709–13.

40. Shimasaki N, Jain A, Campana D. NK cells for cancer immunotherapy. Nat Rev Drug Discov 2020;19:200–18.

41. Gwalani LA, Orange JS. Single degranulations in NK cells can mediate target cell killing. J Immunol 2018;200(9):3231–43.

42. Adams NM, Geary CD, Santosa EK, et al. Cytomegalovirus infection drives avidity selection of natural killer cells. Immunity 2019;50:1381–90.e5.

43. Fujisaki H, Kakuda H, Imai C, et al. Replicative potential of human natural killer cells. Br J Haematol 2009;145:606–13.

44. Mehta RS, Randolph B, Daher M, et al. NK cell therapy for hematologic malignancies. Int J Hematol 2018;107:262–70.

45. Shilling HG, Young N, Guethlein LA, et al. J Immunol 2002;169(1):239–47.

46. Pérez-Martínez A, de Prada Vicente I, Fernández L, et al. Killer cells can exert a graft-vs-tumor effect in haploidentical stem cell transplantation for pediatric solid tumors. Exp Hematol 2012;40(11):882–91.

47. Rouce RH, Sekine T, Weber G, et al. Natural killer cells in pediatric acute lymphoblastic leukemia patients at diagnosis demonstrate an inhibitory phenotype and reduced cytolytic capacity. Blood 2013;122(21):1397.

48. Simonetta F, Alvarez M, Negrin RS. Natural killer cells in graft-versus-host-disease after allogeneic hematopoietic cell transplantation. Front Immunol 2017;8:465.

49. Bachanova V, Cooley S, Defor TE, et al. Clearance of acute myeloid leukemia by haploidentical natural killer cells is improved using IL-2 diphtheria toxin fusion protein. Blood 2014;123(25):3855–63.

50. Miller JS, Soignier Y, Panoskaltsis-Mortari A, et al. Successful adoptive transfer and in vivo expansion of human haploidentical NK cells in patients with cancer. Blood 2005;105(8):3051–7.

51. Ciurea SO, Schafer JR, Bassett R, et al. Phase 1 clinical trial using mbIL21 ex vivo-expanded donor-derived NK cells after haploidentical transplantation. Blood 2017;130(16):1857–68.

52. Boyiadzis M, Agha M, Redner RL, et al. 1 clinical trial of adoptive immunotherapy using "off-the-shelf" activated natural killer cells in patients with refractory and relapsed acute myeloid leukemia. Cytotherapy 2017;19(10):1225–32.

53. Felices M, Lenvik TR, Davis ZB, et al. Generation of BiKEs and TriKEs to Improve NK cell-mediated targeting of tumor cells. Methods Mol Biol 2016;1441:333–46.

54. Kaynar L, Demir K, Turak EE, et al. TcRαβ-depleted haploidentical transplantation results in adult acute leukemia patients. Hematology 2017;22(3):136–44.

55. Reisner Y, Kapoor N, Kirkpatrick D, et al. Transplantation for acute leukaemia with HLA-A and B nonidentical parental marrow cells fractionated with soybean agglutinin and sheep red blood cells. Lancet 1981;2:327–31.

56. Reisner Y, Kapoor N, Kirkpatrick D, et al. Transplantation for severe combined immunodeficiency with HLA-A, B, D, DR incompatible parental marrow cells fractionated by soybean agglutinin and sheep red blood cells. Blood 1983;61:341–8.

57. Aversa F, Tabilio A, Terenzi A, et al. Successful engraftment of T-cell-depleted haploidentical "three-loci" incompatible transplants in leukemia patients by addition of recombinant human granulocyte colony-stimulating factor-mobilized peripheral blood progenitor cells to bone marrow inoculum. Blood 1994;84(11):3948–55.

58. Aversa F, Tabilio A, Velardi A, et al. Treatment of high-risk acute leukemia with T-cell-depleted stem cells from related donors with one fully mismatched HLA haplotype. N Engl J Med 1998;339:1186–93.

59. Lang P, Feuchtinger T, Teltschik HM, et al. Improved immune recovery after transplantation of TCRαβ/CD19-depleted allografts from haploidentical donors in pediatric patients. Bone Marrow Transplant 2015;50(Suppl. 2):S6–10.

60. Chaleff S, Otto M, Barfield RC, et al. A large-scale method for the selective depletion of alphabeta T lymphocytes from PBSC for allogeneic transplantation. Cytotherapy 2007;9(8):746–54.

61. Perko R, Kang G, Sunkara A, et al. Gamma delta T cell reconstitution is associated with fewer infections and improved event-free survival after hematopoietic stem cell transplantation for pediatric leukemia. Biol Blood Marrow Transplant 2015;21(1):130–6.

62. Shelikhova L, Ilushina M, Shekhovtsova Z, et al. αβ T cell-depleted haploidentical hematopoietic stem cell transplantation without antithymocyte globulin in children with chemorefractory acute myelogenous leukemia. Biol Blood Marrow Transplant 2019;25(5):e179–82.

63. Ismail AS, Behrendt CL, Hooper LV, et al. Reciprocal interactions between commensal bacteria and γδ intraepithelial lymphocytes during mucosal injury. J Immunol 2009;182(5):3047.

64. Center for Biologics Evaluation and Research. Cellular and gene therapy guidances. U.S. Food and Drug Administration. Available at: https://www.fda.gov/vaccines-blood-biologics/biologics-guidances/cellular-gene-therapy-guidances. Accessed August 16, 2020.

65. Warkentin PI. Foundation for the accreditation of cellular therapy. Voluntary accreditation of cellular therapies: Foundation for the Accreditation of Cellular Therapy (FACT). Cytotherapy 2003;5(4):299–305.

66. Foundation for the accreditation of cellular therapy. FACT. Available at: http://www.factwebsite.org/Standards/. Accessed August 16, 2020.

67. Foundation for the Accreditation of Cellular Therapy and Joint Accreditation Committee. International standards for hematopoietic cellular therapy product collection, processing, and administration (Seventh edition version 7.0). 2018. Available at: http://www.factwebsite.org/ctstandards/. Accessed August 10, 2020.

68. Foundation for the Accreditation of Cellular Therapy and Joint Accreditation Committee. Common standards for cellular therapies (Second edition). 2019. Available at: http://www.factwebsite.org/commonstandards/. Accessed August 10, 2020.

69. Foundation for the Accreditation of Cellular Therapy and Joint Accreditation. Standards for immune effector cells (first edition version 1.1). 2018. Available at: http://www.factwebsite.org/iecstandards/. Accessed August 10, 2020.

Hemolytic Disease of the Fetus and Newborn
Historical and Current State

Melanie E. Jackson, MBBS, BSc, DCH[a],
Jillian M. Baker, MD, MSc, FRCPC[a,b,c,*]

KEYWORDS

- Hemolytic disease of the fetus and newborn (HDFN) • Rhesus disease (RhD-HDFN)
- Severe hyperbilirubinemia • Neonatal anemia • Neonatal hematology

KEY POINTS

- Hemolytic disease of the fetus and newborn (HDFN) remains prevalent and relevant in neonatal hematology.
- HDFN can cause a spectrum of severity from self-limiting mild morbidity to severe life-threatening disease.
- Rhesus antigen D (RhD) prophylaxis against sensitization has drastically reduced rhesus-HDFN–associated morbidity and mortality.
- Neonatal medicine has improved the supportive management of HDFN and thus reduced the incidence of poor neurologic outcomes.
- There is a global inequality of resources, and thus outcomes, for patients with HDFN.

INTRODUCTION

Hemolytic disease of the fetus and newborn (HDFN) is a potentially life-threatening illness of neonates, caused by maternal-fetal red blood cell antigen incompatibilities. The clinical presentation and natural history are heterogeneous, and range from mildly symptomatic neonates with self-limiting postnatal jaundice to hydrops fetalis and perinatal mortality, including stillbirth. Throughout the last century, there were a significant amount of resources and efforts to ensure the development and maintenance of programs to effectively treat and prevent a large proportion of the morbidity and mortality associated with this disease. However, this problem is far from obsolete.

[a] The Hospital for Sick Children, 555 University Avenue, Toronto, Ontario M5G1X8, Canada; [b] Unity Health Toronto (St. Michael's Hospital), 61 Queen Street East, 2nd, Floor, Toronto, Ontario M5C2T2, Canada; [c] University of Toronto, 27 King's College Circle, Toronto, Ontario M5S 1A1, Canada
* Corresponding author. Unity Health Toronto (St Michael's Hospital), 61 Queen Street East, 2nd, Floor, Toronto, Ontario M5C2T2, Canada.
E-mail address: bakerji@smh.ca

Clin Lab Med 41 (2021) 133–151
https://doi.org/10.1016/j.cll.2020.10.009
0272-2712/21/© 2020 Elsevier Inc. All rights reserved.

The most recognized and often severe form of HDFN is that of rhesus (Rh) disease or Rh antigen D (RhD) HDFN (Rh-HDFN or Rh-HDN), caused by maternal antigens to RhD. Historically, Rh disease has caused most of the perinatal morbidity and mortality from HDFN. Thus, the discovery of a means to provide simple and effective prophylaxis against this condition revolutionized the perinatal outcomes and impact of this disease throughout the twentieth and into the twenty-first century. However, most cases of HDFN are not preventable in the same way and are not always able to be predicted. Therefore, careful antenatal and postnatal care and monitoring are required to manage such cases successfully. Effective perinatal care requires adequate education, knowledge, investigation, and management options, as well as access to therapy and resources, including transfusion and blood products.

HDFN remains a significant cause of worldwide perinatal morbidity as well as ongoing high rates of mortality in many parts of the world despite improvement in Rh-HDFN preventive measures (the most severe type of HDFN), to which there is inequitable access globally. HDFN continues to pose a large burden of disease to health care systems internationally. Ongoing focus on HDFN is required to maintain and improve prevention and mitigate poor outcomes. Health care providers in primary and specialty care have a valuable role to play in providing prompt, evidence-based diagnosis, prevention, investigation, and management to at-risk pregnancies and neonates.

HISTORY

A French midwife reported the first known documented case of HDFN in 1609, describing twins, 1 of whom died of hydrops on day 1 of life, and the other died on day 3 of life after developing severe jaundice and kernicterus.[1] From then until the end of the nineteenth century, approximately 70 reports of similar descriptions were seen in the literature.[2] It was not until 3 centuries after the first case was described that these symptoms and cases were linked together as part of the same disease process. In 1932, it was elucidated that severe hemolysis and extramedullary erythropoiesis lead to hydrops fetalis, postnatal jaundice, and consequent kernicterus; however, the cause was still not understood.[3] Further research led to the accurate theory that maternal antibodies to fetal red blood cells cross the placenta and cause hemolysis.[4] Initially, in 1938, the antibodies were inaccurately postulated to be toward fetal hemoglobin.[5]

Soon after this, in 1940, the Rh blood group system was defined by Landsteiner and Wiener,[7] and the pathogenesis of HDFN became much clearer.[6,7]

There are suggestions that HDFN was at least vaguely identified a long time before any of these instances in the history of the English monarchy and that HDFN may have led to the events that triggered the English Reformation in the sixteenth century.[8] In 1509, Katherine of Aragon married Henry VIII, and subsequently they had 6 children, 5 of whom died in utero or in early infancy.[8] There was only 1 surviving girl, and, because of the perceived lack of ability of produce a live male heir, Henry VIII sought an annulment of the marriage. There were conflicts with the Pope over this request, and the marriage was annulled by the Archbishop of Canterbury, subsequently resulting in the English split from Rome. If the deaths of these offspring were caused by HDFN, as postulated by Rosse[9], HDFN has significantly shaped English and Roman history, and thus the world today.[8]

Some investigators even argue that the description of HDFN in the medical literature extends much earlier than these times. Hippocrates, often referred to as the Father of Medicine, described a condition called fetus carnosus, which is thought by medical historians to have represented fetal hydrops as early as 400 BC.[10,11]

It was not until 1940 that Karl Landsteiner, an Austrian physician and immunologist, and Alexander Wiener, an American immunohematologist, discovered and described the Rh blood group system, in addition to the previously described ABO system, by immunizing cells of guinea pigs and rabbits.[6,7] In 1941, Philip Levine, another American immunohematologist, showed that the RhD antigen was the immune target to the immunoglobulin (Ig) G response seen in erythroblastosis fetalis and showed the ability of the antibody to cross the placenta.[12,13] This work led to the understanding of Rh-HDFN but also the physiologic understanding of how all types of HDFN occur.

Levine continued his work in this area, and in 1956 he showed that the risk of sensitization to the RhD antigen is decreased if the fetus is also ABO incompatible to the mother and the mother has type O blood group.[14] Any fetal cells that enter the maternal circulation are rapidly hemolyzed by the potent and innate maternal anti-A and/or anti-B antibodies, thus reducing the likelihood of maternal exposure to the RhD antigen and subsequent sensitization.[15,16]

In 1961, Ronald Finn, an English medical researcher, made 2 important revelations. He showed that fetal red blood cells circulate in the maternal system in RhD-negative mothers; in fact, in all mothers.[17] He then went on to show that administration of passive anti-D immunoglobulin (Ig) G accelerated the clearance of RhD-positive red blood cells administered to RhD-negative male volunteers. In 1963, Vincent Freda, an American obstetrician, produced the first specific anti-D immunoglobulin preparation.[18,19] In the same year, Schneider,[20] a German physician, was able to show similar results in nonpregnant RhD-negative female volunteers who were given passive anti-D to protect against immunization after infusion of RhD-positive cells.[19] This work has formed the basis of the prevention of sensitization in pregnant women and has saved millions of lives around the world since this discovery.

Although there has been no immunologic development of prophylaxis for other types of HDFN, other advances in neonatal medicine over the last century have led to the increased survival and reduced long-term morbidity of babies born with all types of HDFN (**Box 1**).

PATHOPHYSIOLOGY

HDFN predominantly occurs when the fetus or neonate inherits a red blood cell antigen from the father that is not present on the mother's red blood cells. More than 50 red blood cell antigens have been identified to cause HDFN.[21] The pathophysiology involves the development of maternal IgG antibodies to these particular red blood cell antigens that travel across the placenta. The maternal antibodies identify and attach to fetal red blood cell antigens and cause alloimmune destruction of fetal and neonatal red blood cells by the splenic macrophages. The timing of hemolysis depends on when in development the red blood cell antigen is expressed on the fetal or the neonatal red blood cell, many of which cause problems antenatally, but some not until the postnatal period.[21]

Other than in the instance of ABO incompatibility, the pathophysiology of HDFN requires previous maternal exposure to antigens not expressed on her red blood cells, thus causing sensitization and development of IgM antibodies. In turn, the immune system makes IgG antibodies that can cross the placenta. Prior antigen exposure causes sensitization and thus activation of this alloimmune response for subsequent exposures.[22] However, ABO HDFN (the most common but often the mildest type of HDFN) does not require prior exposure to foreign antibodies because the immune system in type O blood group women naturally develops innate anti-A and anti-B IgG.[22] Note that type A and B group patients also develop the respective antibodies to the

---

Box 1
Timeline of the major advances in hemolytic disease of the fetus and newborn leading to its current management and development

400 BC: Hippocrates described fetus carnosus (likely to be hydrops fetalis)

1609: Louise Bourgeois described twins with HDFN

Seventeenth to nineteenth century: ~70 further cases of likely HDFN described in medical literature

1892: Basic pathogenesis of hydrops fetalis described by Ballantyne

1901: Landsteiner described ABO blood group system

1912: First neonatal red blood cell transfusion

1932: Diamond and colleagues[3] described the link between fetal extramedullary hematopoiesis, jaundice, and kernicterus

1938: Darrow[4] described maternal antibodies in pregnancy and antigen-antibody complexes

1940: Landsteiner and Weiner[7] described Rh blood group system

1941: Levine identifies RhD as immune target during pregnancy and sensitization

1946: Wallerstein[89] introduced neonatal exchange transfusion

1956: Stern and colleagues[15] described coexistent ABO incompatibility as protective for Rh sensitization

1957: Kleihauer[104] described investigation of fetal red blood cells in maternal samples

1958: Cremer introduced phototherapy to neonatal medicine for management of jaundice

1961: Finn and colleagues[17] confirmed that fetal red blood cells circulate in maternal blood circulation

1961: Finn and colleagues[17] showed that passive RhD IgG (anti-D) accelerates removal of RhD-positive cells in RhD-negative pregnant mothers

1963: Freda produced first RhD IgG (anti-D) preparation

1965: Freda and Clarke independently reported success of RhD IgG (anti-D) in preventing RhD sensitization

1968: RhD IgG (anti-D) was first licensed in North America (July)

2018: 50th anniversary of RhD IgG (anti-D) availability; millions of lives saved over 50 years because of this development

---

antigens they do not possess, but they are not normally at risk of HDFN because these antibodies are almost always IgM and do not cross the placenta.[22]

A variety of sensitizing events can lead to the development of causative antibodies, including a previous pregnancy resulting in normal delivery, previous ectopic pregnancy, miscarriage, termination of pregnancy, invasive prenatal diagnostic procedures, fetomaternal hemorrhage (such as that from trauma, external cephalic version, antepartum hemorrhage), as well as previous blood product transfusion and previous exposure of foreign blood products via other means, such as contaminated needles.[23] Sensitization rarely occurs before the first pregnancy. With the exclusion of ABO incompatibility, because most of these sensitization events are pregnancy related, HDFN rarely affects the first pregnancy and often worsens with subsequent pregnancies because of increased sensitization. In some instances, the sensitization event cannot be identified, and it is expected that, in many of these instances, there has been an unidentified miscarriage.[24]

Hemolysis occurs when the macrophages of the reticuloendothelial system, predominantly the spleen and liver, identify the antigen-antibody immune complexes and destroy the cells.[22] Consequently, the fetus compensates for this red blood cell destruction by extramedullary hematopoiesis and produces more red blood cells. If the red blood cell destruction is mild, extramedullary hematopoiesis in the liver and spleen may compensate appropriately. If the red blood cell destruction is severe, there will be severe anemia and multiorgan hypoxia from the reduced ability to deliver oxygen and nutrients adequately, resulting in circulatory and hepatic failure. Liver failure causes decreased protein levels and a reduction in oncotic pressure in the circulation, and heart failure causes an increase in venous pressure; the combination of these leads to generalized edema and ascites, known as hydrops fetalis, which has a high perinatal mortality. Lesser degrees of edema also occur. Erythroblastosis fetalis is a term developed by Rautmer for this condition in 1912.[25] This term refers to hemolysis caused by HDFN in the fetus with subsequent sequelae of hydrops, anemia, and neonatal hyperbilirubinemia.

The severity of hemolysis and disease that each infant develops with HDFN varies greatly.[26] Patients with mild disease may have self-limiting hemolysis and jaundice in the neonatal period, with or without anemia, which may require treatment with phototherapy and red blood cell transfusions. Moderate disease occurs in those patients who develop concerningly high levels of bilirubinemia and thus require exchange transfusion in the neonatal period to prevent neurologic damage. Patients with severe disease often present with fetalis hydrops, diagnosed before or after delivery, which has a high incidence of mortality and morbidity.[22] If these patients are identified early, they may receive intrauterine transfusions.

The antigen to which the antibody develops often dictates the severity of the hemolysis and the disease process. There are 360 red blood cell antigens currently described, divided into 38 grouping systems, with some not allocated a group.[25] This number is increasing with time, because research is revealing newly described antigens. Blood group antigens are typically glycoproteins, and their antigen specificity is established by the oligosaccharide or amino acid sequence. The severity of HDFN varies depending on the immunogenicity of the antigen and antibody complex involved (**Table 1**). In rare instances of HDFN, the antigen is not found.

Maternal antibodies that develop to fetal red blood cell antigens and cross the placenta usually clear the neonate's circulation within 12 weeks.[27] However, it is common for these antibodies to still be present at 6 months in small amounts, albeit without clinically significant hemolysis.[28]

Neonatal hyperbilirubinemia is caused by the destruction of red blood cells and the resulting release of bilirubin. It does not occur before birth because the bilirubin from the red blood cell destruction crosses the placenta and is cleared by the maternal liver. Once the baby is born, the neonate's liver is responsible for processing and excreting the unconjugated bilirubin. The newborn liver is immature and thus produces smaller amounts of the enzyme uridine diphosphate glucuronosyltransferase (UGT).[28] All newborns are at risk for the development of jaundice, because of the natural destruction of fetal hemoglobin; however, those with increased hemolysis caused by HDFN are at risk for higher bilirubin levels. The degree of hemolysis from HDFN and thus hyperbilirubinemia in the postnatal period can lead to severe bilirubin encephalopathy, known as kernicterus.[29] This condition can cause irreversible central neurologic impairment and death for the neonate.

In most forms of HDFN, erythropoiesis is increased in order to compensate for the hemolysis.[30] This process does not occur with Kell blood group alloimmunization because anti-Kell antibodies also suppress erythropoiesis via destruction of

Table 1
Red cell antigens that cause hemolytic disease of the fetus and newborn

Mild HDFN	Moderate HDFN	Severe HDFN
ABO (A, B)	Rh (EW, hrs, Tar, Rh32, HrBE, Hr$_o$)	Rh (D, c, f, Ce, C^w, cE)
Rh (C, e, C^x, VS, CE, Be^a, JAL)	Diego (Di^a, Di^b, Wr^a, ELO)	Kell (K, k, Ku, Js^b)
Kell (Kp^a, Js^a, Ul^a)	Duffy (Fy^a)	Globoside (PP$_1$P$_k$)
Junior (Jra)	Gerbich (Ge3)	MNSs (Vw, Mur, MUT)
Kidd (Jk^a, Jk^b, Jk3)	H (H)	Mittenberger (Mi^a)
Duffy (Fy^b)	Kell (K, k, Ku, Js^b)	MNSs (Vw, Mur, MUT)
Langereis (Lan)	MNSs (U, Ss S, s, Mt^a, M^v)	Gerbich (PP1Pk)
MNSs (M, N, Hil, Or)	Colton (Co^a)	(HJK)
Colton (Co^b, Co^3)	(Kg)	—
Scianna (Rd, SC2)	(Sara)	—
Xg (Xg^a)	—	—
(At^a)	—	—

*System (antigen). Note that some antigens have no system as per International Society of Blood Transfusion classification.
**Classified in usual severity of antigen; variations are described.
***Mild HDFN = published reports needing phototherapy for postnatal jaundice. Moderate HDFN = published reports of needing postnatal exchange transfusion. Severe HDFN = published reports of hydrops fetalis or intrauterine transfusions.

red blood cell progenitor and precursor cells in the bone marrow.[31] Thus, anti-Kell antibodies lead to earlier and more severe anemia than many other alloantibodies and are generally considered to be the most severe type of HDFN after Rh disease.[32]

In the setting of Rh-HDFN, infants born to sensitized mothers, with only mild or no apparent signs and symptoms, can develop late-onset hemolytic disease, which may cause severe hyperbilirubinemia and anemia several weeks into life, showing the need for follow-up beyond the first few days of life for infants known to be at risk.[33]

Some patients have RhD variants. These variants include weak RhD antigens and partial RhD antigens.[34] Patients who have an RhD variant may either have fewer RhD antigenic sites on their red blood cells (weak RhD antigen, previously known as D^u) or they may be missing portions of the antigen (partial RhD antigen, of which there are more than 30 identified types). Variant RhD testing is routinely undertaken for blood donors but is not recommended for prenatal testing in most settings. Patients with weak RhD antigen expression are not prone to alloimmune anti-D sensitization and thus can be safely treated as if they are RhD positive, and, as such, can be transfused with RhD-positive red blood cells.[35] However, patients with partial D can still become alloimmunized and create antibodies to the standard Rh D antigen, and thus need to be managed as RhD-negative individuals. Weak D and partial D show variable results on serologic testing and cannot accurately be typed this way.[34] However, serologic tests with commercial anti-D typically identify partial D variants as RhD negative, so they are treated this way.[34] Molecular genetics of the RhD gene on chromosome 1 is required to accurately differentiate between partial and weak D variants and accurately type the patient. Molecular genetics is suggested when there is a weak serologic response to RhD.[34]

EPIDEMIOLOGY

The true worldwide extent of perinatal morbidity and mortality associated with HDFN is not known.[34] The incidence of each type of HDFN varies substantially among different ethnic groups, depending on the prevalence of the causative red blood cell antigens.[36] The incidence in low-income and middle-income countries is less known, because of a lack of accurate data collection and resources despite the perinatal burden of disease being higher.[22,36]

Rhesus Antigen D Hemolytic Disease of the Fetus and Newborn

Before 1945, before the introduction of effective prevention and management strategies, the perinatal mortality in high-income white countries was approximately 4000 per 100,000 births, and approximately 10% of this estimate was associated with Rh hemolytic disease, which equates to approximately 0.4% of births.[14] Approximately 1% of pregnancies were affected by RhD-HDFN, and an estimated 40% to 50% of these pregnancies resulted in stillbirth or neonatal death.[37,38] The introduction in particular of exchange transfusion as well of prevention of RhD sensitization has dramatically reduced this incidence and mortality.[39]

Differences in the incidence of Rh disease among ethnicities occur because of genetic differences in the prevalence of the RhD gene and differences in population sizes. In white people, approximately 15% of the population is RhD negative, whereas in African populations this figure is 5%, in Chinese populations it is 0.5%, and in Indian populations it is 7%[40]; however, in China, for example, there is a large population and thus the burden of disease is still high despite the low prevalence of RhD-negative individuals.

ABO Hemolytic Disease of the Fetus and Newborn

ABO HDFN is the most common form of HDFN and the leading cause of neonatal jaundice.[41] It almost entirely occurs in type O blood group mothers who have a baby that is type A, B, or AB blood group; however, it can occur in rare circumstances with type A or B group mothers.[42] Consequential anemia and hydrops fetalis are very rare; however, neonatal hyperbilirubinemia is common. ABO incompatibility occurs in 12% to 15% of pregnancies, with evidence of sensitization in approximately 3% to 4% of these pregnancies, as shown by a positive direct Coombs test; however, less than 1% have symptomatic hemolysis.[43]

Other Types of Hemolytic Disease of the Fetus and Newborn

More than 50 other red blood cell antigens have been described to trigger HDFN.[21] Rh antigens other than RhD are often responsible, including the c, C, E, and e antigens.[44] Red blood cell antigens from other groups known to cause severe hemolytic disease include antigens from Kell, Duffy, MNS, Kidd, and P blood group systems (see **Table 1**).[45]

HISTORY OF TREATMENT

Before 1945, when up to 50% of fetuses with Rh-HDFN died, there was no antenatal diagnosis or management of HDFN. The next 2 decades saw great change in the understanding and management of this disease, with advances that are relied on to this day.

With the newly discovered understanding of HDFN in the 1940s by Landsteiner and Wiener,[7] American physician Henry Wallerstein[39] in 1946 introduced the practice of neonatal exchange transfusion. He discovered that exchanging the affected neonate's blood with fresh donor blood could be used to treat and prevent the adverse outcome of kernicterus caused by accumulation of toxic bilirubin from increased hemolysis.[39]

This discovery led to a dramatic decrease in neonatal mortality associated with HDFN by the early 1960s, from 10% to 2% to 3%[46] The prevention of RhD sensitization, and thus prevention of hemolysis, became the focus of therapy for those at risk of Rh-HDFN.

Management of HDFN caused by non-RhD antigens has advanced over time with the advancement in antenatal and neonatal care, including advances in medicine such as management of jaundice, kernicterus, and transfusion.

Development of Rhesus Antigen D Immunoglobulin G

In the mid-1900s, following the discovery of the blood group system and the subsequent understanding of HDFN, 2 physicians separately reported the successful prevention of RhD sensitization by the postpartum administration of passive RhD IgG (also known as anti-D) to RhD-negative mothers with RhD-positive babies. Specifically, in 1965, both Cyril Clarke and Vincent Freda independently reported the successful prevention of RhD sensitization by the postpartum administration of RhD IgG to RhD-negative mothers with RhD-positive babies (see **Box 1**).[14,46,47]

In May of 1968, the first RhD immune globulin treatment introduced by Ortho Clinical Diagnostics (part of Jskymed), was administered to a patient by the name of Marianne Cummins in Teaneck, New Jersey.[48–50] The treatment successfully prevented sensitization in Marianne, and thus risk of HDFN in her future pregnancies. In July 1968, Rh IgG was licensed in North America for use in postpartum women to prevent Rh-HDFN.[38,48] RhD IgG is most commonly given intramuscularly, with minimal side effects including fever and local discomfort or pain.[49]

Prophylactic RhD IgG is the current mainstay treatment to prevent hydrops fetalis and other manifestations of Rh-HDFN, but the exact mechanism of how passive IgG anti-D administration suppresses RhD sensitization is not entirely understood.[51]

This breakthrough in medicine is still viewed as the most successful application of antibody-mediated immunosuppression in history and has recently had its 50th anniversary of mainstream clinical use.[52] To this day, RhD IgG (anti-D) is prepared by pooled human plasma and is used prophylactically both antenatally and postnatally to prevent Rh-HDFN. Initially it was given only postnatally, with further prevention being established with antenatal administration in the 1970s.[53,54] This current regime (where RhD IgG is available) of giving pregnant RhD-negative women a dose of RhD IgG at 28 weeks' gestation and a second dose within 72 hours of the birth of an RhD-negative baby is estimated to have reduced the burden of Rh-HDFN disease by about 95% over the past 52 years.[47]

Because RhD IgG remains a plasma-derived product with the theoretic risk of infectious disease transmission, much research has explored a recombinant option using monoclonal antibodies, particularly in response to the risk of variant Creutzfeldt-Jakob disease.[38,53] Because of several complications, including severe hemolysis, low bioavailability, and other difficulties, these recombinant options have not yet had major success; however, research is ongoing.[38,47]

Prevention of sensitization still relies on blood donors with natural anti-D, identified usually via blood donations. Male donors are generally used and are reexposed periodically to small amounts of the RhD antigen. The donor's immune system creates anti-D antibodies that are collected with plasma donation and then processed. Most countries have a small number of donors who repeatedly donate.[55,56] Adequate donors are generally limited and thus a lot of work is required to identify donors and encourage ongoing, regular plasma donations.

Prevention of Sensitization to Rhesus Antigen D

In the event of a sensitizing event, such as a miscarriage or fetomaternal hemorrhage, RhD IgG (anti-D) should be promptly administered, ideally within 72 hours of the event to successfully prevent sensitization.[57]

Routine RhD IgG is given in North America at 28 weeks, based on the evidence that 92% of people who become sensitized do so after 28 weeks, and it generally lasts 12 weeks and has a half-life of 21 to 24 days.[58,59] It is then repeated after delivery. Different countries have different routine anti-D administration protocols, many also giving a dose at 34 weeks.

Pregnant women with weak RhD variant are treated as if they are RhD positive, and thus do not need to receive anti-D; however, it does not cause harm if they are given anti-D prophylaxis.[34] By contrast, those who have partial D (identified by molecular genetic testing) should be treated as RhD negative, and receive anti-D as clinically indicated in pregnancy, because of the previously described risk of alloimmunization.[60] The most recent American College of Obstetricians and Gynecologists (ACOG) guidelines support these recommendations.[61]

Antibody formation occurs in 1.5% of pregnancies of RhD-negative women carrying an RhD-positive fetus despite adequate prophylaxis.[62] These neonates thus need monitoring and management for potential severe HDFN.

Postpartum Rhesus Antigen D Immunoglobulin G

Postpartum anti-D was first introduced as prophylaxis before the addition of antenatal prophylaxis.[53] It has been globally accepted that the most appropriate standard of care is to administer 300 µg of anti-D.[63] If there is a larger-than-expected fetomaternal hemorrhage preceding or during labor, a larger dose is required to guarantee a reduction in the risk of sensitization. Whether a routine Kleihauer-Betke test to estimate fetamaternal hemorrhage and guide dosing is effective in routine scenarios has been explored, and the conclusions are that this is not cost-effective in scenarios outside of unexpected blood loss.[64]

CURRENT MANAGEMENT

Modern advances in medicine have led to the development of sophisticated obstetric and neonatal units in medium-income to high-income countries, which are able to manage complicated neonatal morbidity and mortality. Advanced antenatal testing and treatment options, including amniotic fluid sampling, fetal blood sampling, and intraperitoneal fetal transfusion, have evolved the management of HDFN, among other technologies.[65] As a consequence, a drastic decrease in the morbidity and mortality from all types of HDFN has occurred.

Antenatal Screening

Routine testing of maternal blood group (ABO and RhD) and antibody screen in the first trimester serves to screen for the risk of HDFN. Antibody screening is typically repeated periodically to screen for newly developed antibodies. Early detection of clinically significant antibodies can allow appropriate additional monitoring for HDFN, as well as other antenatal management options, including transfusion and early delivery.

Maternal antibody titers are performed if there is a positive IgG antibody screen, with an IgG antibody known to be associated with HDFN. Specific antibodies have certain titers (which vary for each antibody), below which HDFN is unlikely and no additional management is required.[66] Measuring titers is also useful for differentiating between passive and immune anti-D; however, the result does not reliably predict the severity of HDFN.[67] Fetal antigen testing is considered if a maternal antibody is greater than the critical titer. Determining the paternal antigen status can help delineate the fetal status; however, this is fraught with potential issues because of the recognized incidence of nonpaternity in society. If the biological father has the antigen corresponding with the antibody, DNA testing can determine homozygosity or heterozygosity. If the father is heterozygous, the fetus may be either positive or negative for the antigen. If homozygous, the fetus is assumed positive.

Fetal DNA testing is available by noninvasive prenatal testing, identifying fetal cells separated from a maternal blood sample.[68] This technology is becoming more readily available worldwide.[69] Alternatively, amniocentesis can provide a sample of fetal cells for DNA sampling. Invasive amniocentesis is often not available and/or not considered a reasonable risk for many expecting mothers and their partners, especially given the risk of fetal loss and even the possibility of enhanced antigen exposure and sensitization. As a lower-risk alternative, ultrasonography can be used to monitor for signs of fetal anemia, specifically looking for increase of the peak velocity in the middle cerebral artery.[70] There is a significant false-positive rate with ultrasonography that may prompt invasive sampling, which can in turn lead to complications.[70]

Prenatal Treatment

Evidence of HDFN is often diagnosed antenatally with routine screening, as described earlier. When found, advances in medicine have allowed effective treatment options of fetal anemia and hydrops, as well as appropriate preparation for delivery of neonates expected to be compromised at birth or thereafter. Prenatal treatment options vary greatly depending on the resources available.

Intrauterine transfusions

When signs of fetal anemia are detected antenatally, intrauterine sampling and subsequently red blood cell transfusions to the fetus can be performed, as first performed in 1963 by Albert Liley[71] in the United States. Initially performed into the intraperitoneal cavity, improved technology and skill has enabled such transfusions directly into the umbilical vein.[72,73] During a single procedure (to minimize risk), fetal hemoglobin and hematocrit levels are performed along with a crossmatch followed by a transfusion with compatible blood. Intrauterine transfusion decreases perinatal death and stillbirths associated with HDFN by 75% to 90%.[74,75]

Prenatal intravenous immunoglobulin

Antenatal intravenous immunoglobulin (IVIg) is sometimes given to RhD-sensitized pregnant women, as well as those sensitized with other red blood cell antigens, to prevent the onset and reduce the severity of hemolytic disease in the fetus and neonate, with variable success. Small studies have shown that early initiation of weekly IVIg therapy at a dose of 1 g/kg at gestational age of 10 to 11 weeks in women with high-titer ($\geq$1:32) maternal RhD antibodies can significantly reduce clinically significant disease, including reducing the need for invasive fetal monitoring, intrauterine transfusion, and postnatal exchange transfusion.[76,77] However, late initiation of this therapy beyond about 16 weeks has not been shown to be effective.[77,78] This therapy is not routinely used, or standardized, across antenatal centers and remains controversial.

Prenatal plasmapheresis

Plasmapheresis or plasma exchange has been used as an option for mothers with positive antibody titers, particularly high titers of antibodies, but is not considered standard of care because of the ambivalence of its effectiveness. This technique in theory removes some of the IgG antibody at risk of crossing the placenta, thus, reducing the degree of HDFN. Ultimately this is intended to reduce the need for invasive fetal testing and management, as well as the postnatal morbidity. It is used variably by different units across the world, and is generally considered to have limited efficacy.[79–81]

Postnatal Treatment

Depending on the severity of the illness at birth and degree of antenatal diagnosis and investigation, babies are born with a broad range of clinical manifestations. Those with hydrops fetalis unmanaged in the antenatal period are likely to need significant supportive therapy, including resuscitation to manage symptomatic anemia and fluid accumulations such as pleural effusions, as well as underdeveloped organs such as pulmonary hypoplasia.

Screening for hemolytic disease of the fetus and newborn

Blood tests are performed postnatally on potentially affected neonates in sensitized pregnancies. This testing includes blood type, hematocrit and hemoglobin levels, direct antiglobulin test (DAT), and serum bilirubin levels. A positive DAT is not specific for HDFN, and a negative DAT does not exclude HDFN. A positive DAT in the absence of abnormal jaundice has a very low positive predictive value.[82] Note that some patients only develop late-onset hemolysis, so, if blood work is initially reassuring, the baby still needs monitoring and clinical assessment for several weeks.[33] This requirement is often forgotten and is thus a cause of preventable morbidity in the current medical environment.[33]

Bilirubin level can be assessed by various means; conventionally, this is done with a blood test to assess the serum bilirubin level, but newer technologies have seen the introduction of transcutaneous monitoring.[83] Transcutaneous sampling is considered to be not as precise, but it serves a purpose in reducing the number of invasive blood samples and in predicting mild to moderately increased bilirubin levels.[81]

Phototherapy

Serum bilirubin concentration can be reduced using phototherapy. Phototherapy uses light of specific wavelengths (450–490 nm).[84] It must be noted that, contrary to some historical teaching and current popular belief, this wavelength is found in natural sunlight, and thus sunlight therapy can be used to treat neonatal jaundice; however, is usually not recommended because of the risk of sunburn.[85,86] The wavelength of the light changes the bilirubin into isomers that are water soluble, and thus performs the role of the underproduced UGT.[84] The kidneys can then excrete the red blood cell destruction byproducts, and the toxic buildup of bilirubin is reduced.[22] This is a slow but effective process. Mild complications of this treatment include bronze skin discoloration, skin rashes, and loose stools.[87] It is common to use phototherapy before and after an exchange transfusion to reduce bilirubin levels.

Most neonatal units have internationally standardized nomograms that guide the use of phototherapy depending on the age of the neonate and the risk of neurologic compromise, many of which internationally use the Bhutani nomogram.[84] Phototherapy can be intensified by increasing the number of lights on the baby, increasing the surface area exposed, and increasing time under the lights. New and novel technologies have been created over the last 30 to 40 years, including biliblankets and bilibeds, which are designed to make phototherapy more practical and effective.[88] A biliblanket uses a fiberoptic light source transmitted via a cable to a fiberoptic mat that delivers a high-intensity, uniform light using a halogen bulb.[88]

Exchange transfusion

Exchange transfusion is used for treatment of HDFN when serum bilirubin levels reach a dangerous level on the nomograms, with high risk of neurologic impairment, including kernicterus. Wallerstein[89] introduced the practice of neonatal exchange transfusion in 1946, and this led to a dramatic reduction in mortality associated with HDFN.

The first exchange transfusion was described in the setting of ABO incompatibility and involved replacing the patient's antibody-coated red blood cells with donated red blood cells, as well as removing the high levels of bilirubin.[86] This procedure remains labor, time, and resource intensive. However, newer automated techniques have reduced the time and labor involved in specialized treatment centers. Regardless, a high level of expertise is required to perform this specialized procedure. Again, it is rare that ABO-incompatibility HDFN causes disease severe enough to require such therapy (see **Table 1**).

Transfusion

Red blood cell transfusion may be required at various stages in the neonatal period. Children born with severe symptomatic anemia need lifesaving transfusion very early in life and sometimes warrant the use of type O RhD-negative donor blood immediately postdelivery. For those not requiring urgent transfusion, hemolysis may lead to the later requirement of a red blood cell transfusion, often within the first few days or weeks of life. As with many elements of neonatal and transfusion medicine, the definition of symptomatic anemia and the hematocrit or hemoglobin level to prompt a red blood cell transfusion vary among treatment facilities, and are often individually tailored to the clinical scenario.

Intravenous immunoglobulin

IVIg is often used in the postnatal period to potentially avoid the necessity for either red blood cell transfusion or exchange transfusion in the neonatal period and remains highly contentious among experts. Although exchange transfusion is an effective treatment, it is invasive, costly, and requires specialized resources and expertise. Other potential side effects of exchange transfusion include electrolyte imbalance such as hypocalcemia, thrombocytopenia, bleeding, thrombosis, and an increased risk of mortality.[90] Ultimately, preventing bilirubin levels necessitating exchange transfusion is in the best interests of the neonate. As such, IVIg has been trialed in HDFN to attempt to halt the increase in bilirubin levels and ideally mitigate the need for an exchange transfusion where possible.[91] A Cochrane Review in 2018 revealed that, although many studies suggest that early postnatal IVIg can effectively reduce the need for both exchange transfusions and the degree of hemolysis, the quality of evidence is low because of inconsistences in treatment thresholds and procedures, variations of management, and lack of blinding.[91] The 2 studies with the highest quality of evidence were subanalyzed and showed no conclusive benefit of using IVIg postnatally to reduce the need for other therapies. IVIg is postulated to be most effective in ABO incompatibility.[8,92,93] However, evidence remains insufficient. Despite the inconclusive evidence, IVIg is incorporated into the care of HDFN in many neonatal treatment centers worldwide, usually in independently guided practice. Recommendations tend to be 0.5 to 1 mg/kg transfused over several hours.[92] Adverse reactions can include iatrogenic hemolysis, especially in group A patients. Importantly, it is considered safe in neonates, despite its high cost.[94]

CURRENT BURDEN OF CARE AND FUTURE DIRECTIONS
High-Income Countries

As previously explained, the incidence of mortality and morbidity from HDFN has greatly decreased, but it is not eradicated even in high-income countries. To maintain the level of care currently provided, donors are needed to provide the huge amount of RhD IgG required, and this demand is increasing. Research continues to investigate synthetic treatment options to reduce this requirement and the unlikely risk of infection from this product. However, alternatives to RhD IgG are not yet an option. Noninvasive prenatal testing of fetal red blood cells is a potential future means of reducing the amount of RhD IgG required, by identifying those fetuses who are RhD negative, and thus anti-D is not required.

It is important that adequate training, resources, and education continue to be provided in high-income countries, despite the reduction in disease burden, because serious cases occur that could have been identified earlier with more vigilant monitoring.[95] Also, there is an increased trend for RhD-negative mothers to refuse RhD immunization because of reluctance and ambivalence about all immunizations, and thus the incidence of preventable Rh-HDFN is increasing again.[96,97]

Worldwide

By contrast, recent evidence confirms that HDFN, including Rh disease, continues to be a public health problem in low-income and middle-income countries, affecting more than 150,000 neonates annually and causing thousands of stillbirths, neonatal deaths, and cases of hyperbilirubinemia with the sequelae of kernicterus and bilirubin-induced neurologic dysfunction.[97–100] In countries without RhD IgG prophylaxis protocols and/or access, as many as 14% of affected fetuses are stillborn and up to 50% of live affected births result in neonatal death or neurologic consequences from HDFN.[22]

The World Health Organization currently recommends antenatal prophylaxis with anti-D immunoglobulin on nonsensitized RhD pregnant women at 28 weeks and 34 weeks of gestation.[101] Many populations do not have access to such testing to determine blood group, let alone provide prophylaxis.[98,99]

HDFN caused by antigens other than RhD are also a problem in such countries. The standard of care in neonatal units is variable and limited because of expense, and many patients cannot access the required care, such as investigations, phototherapy, transfusions, and follow-up care to manage HDFN postnatally.

The future of HDFN in these parts of the world includes exploring ways to compensate for the expense of treatment and includes point-of-care blood group testing, such as Eldon card point-of-care blood grouping (manufactured by Eldon Biologicals). This technique allows inexpensive screening of the blood group in the antenatal setting to identify Rh-negative mothers.[102,103] Also, filtered sunlight trials are being attempted in low-income countries such as Nigeria to allow access to simple and cheap postnatal therapy in the place of standard phototherapy.[86]

SUMMARY

The prevention and management of HDFN has been revolutionized in the last century, reducing the previously substantial degree of morbidity and mortality to a minimum. RhD immunoglobulin treatment, recently having its 50th anniversary, is considered one of the most successful breakthroughs in medicine over the last century. However, HDFN remains a pertinent part of neonatal medicine, with management relying on blood banking techniques, blood products, and transfusions for life-saving management, as well as sophisticated antenatal and neonatal care.

Although modern medicine has significantly improved outcomes, like many other diseases there remains a huge gap in care between high-income and low-income countries. Ongoing advances in medicine are needed to make prevention and treatment available in an equitable way worldwide. Transfusion medicine and blood banking have been pertinent to the advances in this area of hematology and neonatology and continue to have a crucial role in the management of HDFN.

DISCLOSURE

The authors have nothing to disclose.

REFERENCES

1. Bourgeois L. Observations diverses sur la stérilité, perte de fruict, foecondité accouchements et maladies des femmes et enfants nouveaux naiz. Am J Obstet Gynecol 1995;173(6):1893–4.
2. Santavy J. Hemolytic disease in the newborn - history and prevention in the world and the Czech republic. Biomed Pap Med Fac Univ Palacky Olomouc Czech Repub 2010;154(2):147–51.
3. Diamond LK, Blackfan KD, Baty JM. Erythroblastosis fetalis and its association with universal edema of the fetus, icterus gravis neonatorum and anemia of the newborn. J Pediatr 1932;1(3):269–309.
4. Darrow RR. Icterus gravis (Erythroblastosis) neonatorum. Rhesus Haemolytic Disease 1938;3–37. https://doi.org/10.1007/978-94-011-6138-1_1.
5. Fasano RM, Hendrickson JE, Luban NLC, Burns MC. Chapter 55: alloimmune hemolytic disease of the fetus and newborn. In: Kaushansky K, Lichtman MA, Prchal JT, et al, editors. Williams hematology. 9th edition. New York (NY): McGraw-Hill Medical; 2010.
6. Kantha SS. The blood revolution initiated by the famous footnote of Karl Landsteiner's 1900 paper. Ceylon Med J 1995;40(3):123–5.
7. Landsteiner K, Wiener AS. An agglutinable factor in human blood recognized by immune sera for rhesus blood. Rhesus Haemolytic Disease 1940;41–2. https://doi.org/10.1007/978-94-011-6138-1_3.
8. Stockman JA. Overview of the state of the art of Rh disease: history, current clinical management, and recent progress. J Pediatr Hematol Oncol 2001;23(8):554–62.
9. Rosse WF. Clinical Immunohematology: Basic Concepts in Clinical Applications. Boston: Blackwell Scientific Publications; 1990.
10. Ballantyne JW. Manual of antenatal pathology and hygiene: the fetus. JAMA 1902;XXXIX(13):783.
11. Ballantyne JW. The Diseases and Deformities of the Foetus. Edinburgh: Oliver and Boyd; 1885.
12. Levine P. Serological Factors as Possible Causes in Spontaneous Abortions. In: Rhesus haemolytic disease. Springer; 1943.
13. Levine P, Katzin EM, Burnham L. Isoimmunization in pregnancy. J Am Med Assoc 1941;116(9):825.
14. Wegmann A, Ghick R. The history of rhesus prophylaxis with anti-D. Eur J Pediatr 1996;155(10):835–8.
15. Stern K, Davidsohn I, Masaitis L. Experimental studies on Rh immunization. Am J Clin Pathol 1956;26(8):833–43.

16. Stern K, Goodman HS, Berger M. Experimental isoimmunization to hemoantigens in man. Rhesus Haemolytic Disease 1961;161–9. https://doi.org/10.1007/978-94-011-6138-1_28.
17. Finn R, Clarke CA, Donohoe WTA, et al. Experimental studies on the prevention of Rh haemolytic disease. BMJ 1961;1(5238):1486–90.
18. Freda VJ, Gorman JG, Pollack W. Successful prevention of experimental Rh sensitization in man with an anti-Rh Gamma2-globulin antibody preparation: a preliminary report. Rhesus Haemolytic Disease 1964;177–84. https://doi.org/10.1007/978-94-011-6138-1_30.
19. Freda V, Gorman J, Pollack W. Prevention of rhesus hæmolytic disease. Lancet 1965;286(7414):690.
20. Schneider J. Die quantitative Bestimmung fetaler Erythrocyten im miitterlichen Kreislauf und deren beschleunigter Abbau durch Antik6rperseren. Geburtshilfe Frauenheilkd 1963;3:562–8.
21. Moise KJ. Hemolytic disease of the fetus and newborn. Clin Adv Hematol Oncol 2013;11(10):664–6.
22. Dror Y, Chan AKC, Baker JM, et al, editors. Hematology avery's neonatology, pathophysiology, and management of the newborn. Wolters Kluwer: Philadelphia; 7th edition.
23. Kumpel BM. On the immunologic basis of Rh immune globulin (anti-D) prophylaxis. Transfusion 2006;46(9):1652–6.
24. Zipursky A, Israels LG. The pathogenesis and prevention of Rh immunization. Rhesus Haemolytic Disease 1967;253–66. https://doi.org/10.1007/978-94-011-6138-1_40.
25. International society of blood transfusion. Available at: https://www.isbtweb.org/working-parties/red-cell-immunogenetics-and-blood-group-terminology/#:~:text=In%201980%20the%20ISBT%20established,use%20of%20a%20specific%20antibody. Accessed August 31, 2020.
26. Dean L. Blood groups and red cell antigens [Internet]. Chapter 4, Hemolytic disease of the newborn. Bethesda (MD): National Center for Biotechnology Information (US); 2005. Available at: https://www.ncbi.nlm.nih.gov/books/NBK2266/.
27. Ross ME, Waldron PE, Cashore WJ, et al. Hemolytic disease of the fetus and newborn. In: de Alacon PA, Werner EJ, Christensen RD, editors. Neonatal hematology: pathogenesis, diagnosis, and management of hematologic problems. 2nd edition. Cambridge (United Kingdom): Cambridge University Press; 2013.
28. Mitchell S, James A. Severe late anemia of hemolytic disease of the newborn. Paediatr Child Health 1999;4(3):201–3.
29. Leung AK, Sauve RS. Breastfeeding and breast milk jaundice. J R Soc Health 1989;109(6):213–7.
30. Gourley GR. Bilirubin metabolism and kernicterus. Adv Pediatr 1997;44:173–229.
31. AU Vaughan JI, Warwick R, Letsky E, et al. Erythropoietic suppression in fetal anemia because of Kell alloimmunization. Am J Obstet Gynecol 1994;171(1):247.
32. de Haas M, Thurik FF, Koelewijn JM, et al. Haemolytic disease of the fetus and newborn. Vox Sang 2015;109(2):99–113.
33. Haider M, Memon S, Tariq F, et al. Rhesus isoimmunization: late-onset hemolytic disease of the newborn without jaundice. Cureus 2020;12(1):e6559.
34. Sandler SG, Chen LN, Flegel WA. Serological weak D phenotypes: a review and guidance for interpreting the RhD blood type using the RHD genotype. Br J Haematol 2017;179(1):10–9.

35. Rizzo C, Castiglia L, Arena E, et al. Weak D and partial D: our experience in daily activity. Blood Transfus 2012;10(2):235–6.
36. Basu S, Kaur R, Kaur G. Hemolytic disease of the fetus and newborn: current trends and perspectives. Asian J Transfus Sci 2011;5(1):3–7.
37. Ree IMC, Smits-Wintjens VEHJ, van der Bom JG, et al. Neonatal management and outcome in alloimmune hemolytic disease. Expert Rev Hematol 2017; 10(7):607–16.
38. Bowman JM. RhD hemolytic disease of the newborn. N Engl J Med 1998; 339(24):1775–7.
39. Wallerstein H. Treatment of severe erythroblastosis by simultaneous removal and replacement of blood of the newborn. Science 1946;103:583–4.
40. Mourant A, Kipec A, Domaniewska-Sobezak K. The distribution of human blood groups and other polymorphisms. London (United Kingdom): Oxford University Press; 1976.
41. Murray NA, Roberts IA. Haemolytic disease of the newborn. Arch Dis Child Fetal Neonatal Ed 2007;92(2):F83–8.
42. Jeon H, Calhoun B, Pothiawala M, et al. Significant ABO hemolytic disease of the newborn in a group B infant with a group A2 mother. Immunohematology 2000;16(3):105–8.
43. McDonnell M, Hannam S, Devane S. Hydrops fetalis due to ABO incompatibility. Arch Dis Child Fetal Neonatal Ed 1998;78:F220–1.
44. Dean L. Blood groups and red cell antigens. Bethesda (MD): National Center for Biotechnology Information (US); 2005. Chapter 7, The Rh blood group. https://www.ncbi.nlm.nih.gov/books/NBK2269/. Available at:.
45. Lopriore E, Rath ME, Liley H, et al. Improving the management and outcome in haemolytic disease of the foetus and newborn. Blood Transfus 2013;11(4): 484–6.
46. Freda VJ, Gorman JG, Pollack W. Successful prevention of experimental Rh sensitisation in man with an anti-Rh gamma-2-globulin preparation: a preliminary report. Transfusion 1964;4:26–32.
47. Weatherall DJ. Cyril Clarke and the prevention of rhesus haemolytic disease of the newborn. Br J Haematol 2012;157:41–6.
48. Bowman J. Thirty-five years of Rh prophylaxis. Transfusion 2003;43:1661–6.
49. Kedrion biopharma inc. RhoGam product label. Available at: https://www2.vaxserve.com/views/PDF/RhoGAM%20Ultra-Filtered%20Plus%20Package%20Insert%207-07.pdf. Accessed August 31, 2020.
50. Silver RM. RhD immune globulin: over 50 years of remarkable progress. BJOG 2016;123(8):1347. https://doi.org/10.1111/1471-0528.13868. Available at:.
51. Kumpel BM, Elson CJ. Mechanism of anti-D-mediated immune suppression–a paradox awaiting resolution? Trends Immunol 2001;22(1):26–31.
52. Hadley AG, Kumpel BM. The role of Rh antibodies in haemolytic disease of the newborn. Baillieres Clin Haematol 1993;6(2):423–44.
53. Liumbruno GM, D'Alessandro A, Rea F, et al. The role of antenatal immunoprophylaxis in the prevention of maternal-foetal anti-Rh(D) alloimmunisation. Blood Transfus 2010;8(1):8–16.
54. Kumpel BM, Saldova R, Koeleman CAM, et al. Anti-D monoclonal antibodies from 23 human and rodent cell lines display diverse IgG Fc-glycosylation profiles that determine their clinical efficacy. Sci Rep 2020;10(1):1464.
55. Harrison James. Australian man with special blood type saves 2 million babies. The huffington post. March 24. 2010. Available at: https://www.huffpost.com/entry/james-harrison-australian_n_512112. Accessed August 31, 2020.

56. Dean M. Wanted: Rh D negative donors. Australian prescriber. 2000. Available at: https://www.nps.org.au/australian-prescriber/articles/wanted-rh-d-negative-donors#. Accessed August 31, 2020.

57. Crowther CA, Middleton P. Anti-D administration after childbirth for preventing Rhesus alloimmunisation. Cochrane Database Syst Rev 1997. https://doi.org/10.1002/14651858.cd000021.

58. Bowman JM. The prevention of Rh immunization. Transfus Med Rev 1988;2(3):129–50.

59. Eklund J, Hermann M, Kjellman H, et al. Turnover rate of anti-D IgG injected during pregnancy. BMJ 1982;284(6319):854–5.

60. Lukacevic Krstic J, Dajak S, Bingulac-Popovic J, et al. Anti-D antibodies in pregnant D variant antigen carriers initially typed as RhD. Transfus Med Hemother 2016;43(6):419–24.

61. Committee on Practice Bulletins-Obstetrics. Practice bulletin No. 181: prevention of Rh D alloimmunization, 130. New York (NY): Obstetrics and Gynecology; 2017. p. e57–70, 1953.

62. Crowther CA, Middleton P, McBain RD. Anti-D administration in pregnancy for preventing Rhesus alloimmunisation. Cochrane Database Syst Rev 2013;2:CD000020.

63. Klein H, Anstee DJ. Haemolytic disease of the fetus and newborn. In: Mollison's blood transfusion in clinical medicine. 11th edition. Oxford (United Kingdom): Blackwell Publishing; 2005. p. 496–545.

64. Mahboob U, Mazhar SB. Role of Kleihauer test in Rhesus negative pregnancy. J Coll Physicians Surg Pak 2006;16(2):120–3.

65. Lindenburg I, T M, van Kamp I L, et al. Intrauterine blood transfusion: current indications and associated risks. Fetal Diagn Ther 2014;36:263–71.

66. Bennardello F, Coluzzi S, Curciarello G, et al. Italian society of transfusion medicine and immunohaematology (SIMTI) and Italian society of gynaecology and obstetrics (SIGO) working group. Recommendations for the prevention and treatment of haemolytic disease of the foetus and newborn. Blood Transfus 2015;13(1):109–34.

67. Gottvall T, Hildén JO. Concentration of anti-D antibodies in Rh(D) alloimmunized pregnant women, as a predictor of anemia and/or hyperbilirubinemia in their newborn infants. Acta Obstet Gynecol Scand 1997;76(8):733–8.

68. Norwitz ER, Levy B. Noninvasive prenatal testing: the future is now. Rev Obstet Gynecol 2013;6(2):48–62.

69. Chandrasekharan S, Minear MA, Hung A, et al. Noninvasive prenatal testing goes global. Sci Transl Med 2014;6(231):231fs15.

70. Shourbagy SE, Elsakhawy M. Prediction of fetal anemia by middle cerebral artery Doppler. Middle East Fertil Soc J 2012;17(4):275–82.

71. Liley AW. Intrauterine transfusion of foetus in haemolytic disease. Br Med J 1963;2(5365):1107–9.

72. Berkowitz RL, Hobbins JC. Intrauterine transfusion utilizing ultrasound. Obstet Gynecol 1981;57:33–6.

73. Pasman SA, Claes L, Lewi L, et al. Intrauterine transfusion for fetal anemia due to red blood cell alloimmunization: 14 years experience in Leuven. Facts Views Vis Obgyn 2015;7(2):129–36.

74. Kanhai HH, Bennebroek Gravenhorst J, Van Kamp IL, et al. Management of severe hemolytic disease with ultrasound-guided intravascular fetal transfusions. Vox Sang 1990;59:180–4.

75. Rodeck CH, Kemp JR, Holman CA, et al. Direct intravascular fetal blood transfusion by fetoscopy in severe Rhesus isoimmunisation. Lancet 1981;1:625–7.

76. Williams D, Argaez C. Off-label use of intravenous immunoglobulin for hematological conditions: a review of clinical effectiveness. Ottawa (ON): Canadian agency for drugs and technologies in health. 2018. Available at: https://www.ncbi.nlm.nih.gov/books/NBK531790/. Accessed August 31, 2020.

77. Mayer B, Hinkson L, Hillebrand W, et al. Efficacy of antenatal intravenous immunoglobulin treatment in pregnancies at high risk due to alloimmunization to red blood cells. Transfus Med Hemother 2018;45(6):429–36.

78. Ambika S, Wong G, Salhotra A, et al. Rekha parameswaran; early intravenous immunoglobulin (IVIG) therapy and non invasive fetal monitoring in rh alloimmunization (AI) and pregnancy. Blood 2008;112(11):4069.

79. Rock G, Lafreniere I, Chan L, et al. Plasma exchange in the treatment of hemolytic disease of the newborn. Transfusion 1981;21:546–51.

80. Maki Y, Ushijima J, Furukawa S, Inagaki H, et al. Plasmapheresis for the treatment of anti-M alloimmunization in pregnancy. Case Rep Obstet Gynecol 2020;2020:9283438.

81. Padmanabhan A, Connelly-Smith L, Aqui N, et al. Guidelines on the use of therapeutic apheresis in clinical practice - evidence-based approach from the writing committee of the American society for apheresis: the eighth special issue. J Clin Apheresis 2019;34(3):171–354.

82. van Rossum HH, de Kraa N, Thomas M, et al. Comparison of the direct antiglobulin test and the eluate technique for diagnosing haemolytic disease of the newborn. Pract Lab Med 2015;3:17–22.

83. Ercan E, Ozg G. The accuracy of transcutaneous bilirubinometer measurements to identify the hyperbilirubinemia in outpatient newborn population. Clin Biochem 2018;55:69–74.

84. Bhutani VK, Stark AR, Lazzeroni LC. Initial clinical testing evaluation and risk assessment for universal screening for hyperbilirubinemia screening group. Predischarge screening for severe neonatal hyperbilirubinemia identifies infants who need phototherapy. J Pediatr 2013;162(3):477–82.

85. Salih FM. Can sunlight replace phototherapy units in the treatment of neonatal jaundice? An in vitro study. Photodermatol Photoimmunol Photomed 2001;17(6):272–7.

86. Slusher TM, Olusanya BO, Vreman HJ, et al. Treatment of neonatal jaundice with filtered sunlight in Nigerian neonates: study protocol of a non-inferiority, randomized controlled trial. Trial 2013;14:446.

87. Wiener AS, Wexler IB, Gamrin E. Hemolytic disease of the fetus and the newborn infants with special reference to transfusion therapy and the use of the biological test for detecting Rh sensitivity. Am J Dis Child 1944;68:317.

88. Donel J. Bili blanket phototherapy. Int J Contemp Pediatr 2019;6(5):2231–4.

89. Wallerstein H. Treatment of severe erythroblastosis fetalis by simultaneous removal and replacement of the blood of the newborn infant. Science 1946;103:583.

90. Jackson JC. Adverse events associated with exchange transfusion in healthy and ill newborns. Pediatrics 1997;99(5):E7.

91. Zwiers C, Scheffer-Rath MEA, Lopriore E, et al. Immunoglobulin for alloimmune hemolytic disease in neonates. Cochrane Database Syst Rev 2018;3. https://doi.org/10.1002/14651858.CD003313.pub2.

92. Beken S, Hirfanoglu I, Turkyilmaz C, et al. Intravenous immunoglobulin G treatment in ABO hemolytic disease of the newborn, is it myth or real? Indian J Hematol Blood Transfus 2014;30(1):12–5.

93. Williams D, Argaez C. Off-label use of intravenous immunoglobulin for hematological conditions: a review of clinical effectiveness . Canadian agency for drugs and technologies in health. 2018. Available at: https://www.ncbi.nlm.nih.gov/books/NBK531790/. Accessed August 31, 2020.

94. Mundy CA, Bhatia J. Immunoglobulin transfusion in hemolytic disease of the newborn: place in therapy. Int J Clin Transfus Med 2015;3:41–5.

95. Baker JM, Campbell DM, Bhutani VK, et al. Rh sensitization in Canada is not obsolete. Paediatr Child Health 2017;22(4):238–9.

96. Pilgrim H, Lloyd-Jones M, Rees A. Routine antenatal anti-D prophylaxis for RhD-negative women: a systematic review and economic evaluation. 2009. In: NIHR Health Technology Assessment programme: Executive Summaries. Southampton (UK): NIHR Journals Library; 2003. Available at: https://www.ncbi.nlm.nih.gov/books/NBK56828/. Accessed August 31, 2020.

97. Zipursky A, Bhutani B. Rhesus disease: a major public health problem. Lancet 2015;386(9994):651.

98. MacKenzie IZ, Findlay J, Thompson K, et al. Compliance with routine antenatal rhesus D prophylaxis and the impact on sensitisations: observations over 14 years. BJOG 2006;113(7):839–43.

99. Zipursky A, Bhutani VK, Odame I. Rhesus disease: a global prevention strategy. Lancet Child Adolesc Health 2018;2(7):536–42.

100. Zipursky A, Paul VK. The global burden of Rh disease. Arch Dis Child Fetal Neonatal Ed 2011;96(2):F84–5.

101. Crowther CA, Keirse MJ. Anti-D administration in pregnancy for preventing rhesus alloimmunisation. Cochrane Database Syst Rev 2000;2:CD000020.

102. Eldon K. Experience with ABO and Rh blood-grouping cards (Eldon cards). Br Med J 1956;2(5003):1218–20.

103. Bienek DR, Charlton DG. Accuracy of user-friendly blood typing kits tested under simulated military field conditions. Mil Med 2011;176(4):454–60.

104. Kleihauer (1974) Determination of Fetal Hemoglobin: Elution Technique, CRC Critical Reviews in Clinical Laboratory Sciences, 5:1, 50-52, DOI: 10.3109/10408367409107625.

Novel Blood Component Therapies in the Pediatric Setting

Shannon C. Walker, MD[a], Jennifer Andrews, MD, MSc[b,c],*

KEYWORDS

- Whole blood • Pathogen-reduced blood products • Pediatrics

KEY POINTS

- There are limited data available on the safety and efficacy of new blood preparation techniques, such as pathogen reduction, and adjuvant therapies, such as fibrinogen concentrate, in children.
- Whole blood, which was historically used more frequently in infants and children undergoing cardiopulmonary bypass surgery, is being used in new clinical scenarios, including trauma resuscitation.
- Prospective, randomized clinical trials in larger numbers of children are needed to further characterize the safety and clinical efficacy of novel blood component therapies, especially because wider use is expected.

INTRODUCTION

The dogma of transfusion medicine for the last several decades has been the use of blood component therapy; that is, packed red blood cells (RBCs), platelets, and plasma and cryoprecipitate for the treatment or prevention of anemia, thrombocytopenia and hypocoagulability or bleeding, and hypofibrinogenemia, respectively. Recently there has been a surge in both new preparation techniques to make existing blood components safer, such as pathogen reduction, and the use of adjuvant treatments, such as fibrinogen concentrate, to prevent bleeding and subsequent use of blood components. Although these newer blood products or blood derivatives have been studied and used more often in adult patients, this article reviews these products

[a] Department of Pediatrics, Division of Hematology/Oncology, Vanderbilt University Medical Center, Preston Research Building #397, 2220 Pierce Avenue, Nashville, TN 37232, USA; [b] Department of Pathology, Microbiology and Immunology, Division of Transfusion Medicine, Vanderbilt University Medical Center, 1301 Medical Center Drive, Suite 4605, Nashville, TN 37232, USA; [c] Department of Pediatrics, Division of Hematology/Oncology, Vanderbilt University Medical Center, 1301 Medical Center Drive, Suite 4605, Nashville, TN 37232, USA
* Corresponding author. Vanderbilt University Medical Center, 1301 Medical Center Drive, Suite 4605, Nashville, TN 37232, USA.
E-mail address: jennifer.andrews@vanderbilt.edu

Clin Lab Med 41 (2021) 153–171
https://doi.org/10.1016/j.cll.2020.10.010
0272-2712/21/© 2020 Elsevier Inc. All rights reserved.

and the existing literature regarding their safety and efficacy in children because their use is likely to become more common:

- Whole blood (WB)
- Solvent/detergent-treated blood products, such as Octoplas
- Pathogen-reduced (PR) blood products, such as INTERCEPT and Mirasol platelet components
- Fibrinogen concentrate

WHOLE BLOOD

WB is not a new product or technique but is the foundation of transfusion medicine that is making a resurgence, especially in trauma resuscitation.[1] WB was initially described in the early 1990s for use in children undergoing complex cardiac surgery, and additional studies of its use in pediatric trauma and other pediatric surgeries have been recently described[2–5] (**Table 1**).

Use in Children Undergoing Cardiac Surgery Requiring Cardiopulmonary Bypass

In 1991, Manno and colleagues,[2] prospectively randomized 161 pediatric patients undergoing open heart surgery that required the use of cardiopulmonary bypass (CPB) and compared 24-hour postoperative blood loss in 52 patients who had postoperative blood transfusions with very fresh whole blood (VFWB) (administered within 6 hours of collection from the blood donor), 57 patients with WB (collected and stored for 24–48 hours), and 52 patients with reconstituted blood component products (RBCs, fresh frozen plasma [FFP], and platelets in a 1:1:1 ratio). WB was used to prime the CPB unit for all patients who were comparable in each treatment arm in age, gender, surgical complexity, mean bypass time, and preoperative coagulation studies. There was no significant difference in the patient groups with respect to the mean amount of blood per kilogram transfused 24 hours postoperatively. However, in the 93 patients less than 2 years of age, 24 hour postoperative blood loss was significantly less in those children who had received either VFWB (mean of 52.3 mL/kg) or WB (mean of 51.7 mL/kg) versus those who had received reconstituted blood component therapy (mean of 96.2 mL/kg) ($P = .001$). The investigators concluded that, for children less than 2 years old undergoing complex open heart surgery, WB, either very fresh or stored for less than 48 hours, was most beneficial in decreasing 24-hour postoperative blood loss.[2] Many pediatric cardiovascular surgeons prefer the use of WB for infants, with 24% of responding pediatric open heart programs surveyed in 2004 in North America reported using WB for CPB.[6]

In 2004, Mou and colleagues[7] compared 96 infants less than 12 months of age who received WB collected within 48 hours for bypass circuit priming before open heart surgery with 104 infants who received reconstituted blood components for CPB priming in a randomized, prospective, double-blinded trial. All infants received standard blood component therapy after this bypass blood priming. The primary outcome, a composite score of survival and length of stay (LOS), did not differ between the groups, although infants who received reconstituted blood components did have shorter LOS (70.5 hours) compared with infants who received WB (97 hours) ($P = .04$). There was no statistical difference in early postoperative chest tube output, transfusion requirements, serum markers of inflammation, cardiac troponin I measurements, and (most importantly) clinical outcomes including death, severe postoperative clinical course, delayed sternal closure, or need for extracorporeal membrane oxygenation between the groups. The investigators concluded that the long-accepted

Table 1
Studies of whole blood use in pediatrics

Reference	Patient Population Studied (n)	Blood Products Compared	Primary Outcome	Secondary Outcomes	Strengths	Caveats
Manno et al,[2] 1991	Children aged 0–20 y undergoing congenital heart surgery with use of CPB (n = 161)	Postoperative transfusions: VFWB (n = 52) vs WB (n = 57) vs RWB (RBCs, FFP, platelets given in a 1:1:1 ratio) (n = 52)	Mean 24-h postoperative blood loss: VFWB: 50.9 mL/kg (SD ± 9.3) WB: 44.8 mL/kg (SD ± 6.0) RWB: 74.2 mL/kg (SD ± 8.9) ($P = .03$)	In patients <2y old, 24-h postoperative blood loss: VFWB: 52.3 mL/kg (SD ± 10.8) WB: 51.7 mL/kg (SD ± 7.4) RWB: 96.2 mL/kg (SD ± 10.7) ($P = .001$)	Prospective, double-blinded, randomized controlled trial	Not truly randomized because parents asked to provide directed donors for children to receive VFWB
Mou et al,[7] 2004	Neonates aged up to 364 d old undergoing congenital heart surgery with use of CPB (n = 200)	CPB bypass prime: FWB (n = 96) vs reconstituted products (RBCs and FFP) (n = 104)	Composite score for survival and LOS in the ICU did not differ	ICU LOS: FWB 97 h vs RBC/FFP 70.5 h ($P = .04$) Cumulative fluid balance: FWB +28.8 mL/kg vs RBC/FFP −6.9 mL/kg ($P = .003$)	Prospective, double-blinded, randomized controlled trial	—
Valleley et al,[8] 2007	Children aged 1 d to 4 y old who underwent cardiac surgery with use of CPB (n = 100)	CPB bypass prime: FWB (n = 61) vs RBC (n = 39)	Donor exposures: 62% of FWB patients had 1 exposure vs 18% of RBC patients ($P<.01$)	No difference in postoperative blood loss	—	Retrospective cohort study. May have been influenced by FWB availability

(continued on next page)

Table 1
(continued)

Reference	Patient Population Studied (n)	Blood Products Compared	Primary Outcome	Secondary Outcomes	Strengths	Caveats
Gruenwald et al,[9] 2008	Neonates aged up to 30 d who required cardiac surgery with use of CPB (n = 64)	CPB bypass prime and 24-h postoperative transfusions: Fresh RWB (n = 31) vs standard blood components (n = 33)	4–24-h postoperative chest tube drainage: RWB 7.7 mL/kg vs standard blood component 11.8 mL/kg (P = .03)	Median hospital LOS: RWB 12 d vs standard 18 d (P = .006) Median total ventilation time RWB 119 h vs standard 164 h (P = .04)	Prospective, randomized controlled trial	Only surgeons were blinded
Jobes et al,[10] 2015	Children <2 y of age who underwent elective cardiac surgery requiring CPB (n = 4111)	CPB bypass prime and immediate postoperative CPB volume replacement: 2 units of WB (n = 3836) vs standard component therapy (n = 252)	WB cohort compared with historical standard components cohort showed decreased donor exposures across multiple areas of cardiac surgery	—	—	Retrospective cohort study; no clinical outcomes compared
Thottathil et al,[5] 2017	Children <4 y of age who underwent complex cranial vault reconstruction surgery (n = 111)	Intraoperative and postoperative transfusion needs: WB (n = 52) or RWB (RBCs/FFP) (n = 59)	62% of WB cohort had ≤1 blood donor exposure compared with 39% in the RWB cohort (P = .02)	No evidence of postoperative coagulopathy in either cohort. No difference in drain blood loss	—	Retrospective cohort study

Leeper et al,[3] 2018	Traumatically injured children >3 y of age weighing more than 15 kg (n = 68)	LTOWB trauma units (n = 18) compared with standard blood products (n = 50)	Median time from admission to transfusion start: WB 15 min vs RBC, plasma, and platelets 303 min ($P<.01$)	No difference in transfusion reactions between groups	Prospective cohort compared with historical controls	No clinical outcomes compared; very small study
Leeper et al,[4] 2019	Traumatically injured children >2 y of age weighing more than 10 kg (n = 22)	LTOWB (n = 8) compared with standard blood components (n = 14)	No difference in posttransfusion platelet counts or platelet function via TEG maximum amplitude	—	Prospective cohort compared with historical controls	No clinical outcomes compared; very small study

Abbreviations: CPB, cardiopulmonary bypass; FFP, fresh frozen plasma; FWB, fresh whole blood; ICU, intensive care unit; LOS, length of stay; LTOWB, low-titer O whole blood; RWB, reconstituted whole blood; SD, standard deviation; TEG, thromboelastography; VFWB, very fresh whole blood; WB, whole blood.

practice of CPB priming with WB did not confer a significant clinical advantage compared with CPB priming with reconstituted blood products.[7]

In 2007, Valleley and colleagues[8] performed a retrospective chart review of 100 children who underwent CPB during cardiac surgery, 61 of whom received WB for CPB priming and 39 of whom received RBCs. Most patients did not receive further transfusions. Postoperative blood loss and clinically relevant postoperative outcomes including death, delayed sternal closure, need for mediastinal reexploration, and extubation were similar between the 2 groups. The investigators concluded that children treated with WB had less donor exposure (62% were exposed to only 1 WB donor) than children treated with RBCs (only 18% were exposed to only 1 blood donor) (P<.001).[8]

In 2008, Gruenwald and colleagues[9] performed a randomized prospective trial comparing 31 neonates less than 1 month of age undergoing cardiac surgery who received reconstituted fresh WB (RBCs, FFP, and platelets collected from the same donor within 2 days of the surgery, processed in the usual manner, and reconstituted just before transfusion) to prime the bypass circuit and for any transfusions in the first 24 hours postoperatively with 33 neonates who received RBCs to prime the bypass circuit and then standard blood component therapy in the first 24 hours postoperatively.[9] There was a significant difference in the primary outcome of the study, chest tube drainage between 4 and 24 hours postoperatively, with the neonates who received reconstituted WB having 7.7 mL/kg of median chest tube loss versus 11.8 mL/kg in those neonates who received standard blood component therapy (P = .03). Median hospital LOS was shorter in surviving neonates who received reconstituted WB (12 days) than in those who received component therapy (18 days) (P = .006). Median total ventilation time or time to first extubation was also significantly less in the reconstituted WB group (119 hours) than in the group who received component therapy (164 hours) (P = .04). Other secondary outcomes (ie, inotrope score and, importantly, transfusion need) were not significantly different. The investigators concluded that neonates receiving reconstituted fresh WB have significantly less chest tube drainage and improved clinical outcomes. They acknowledged that the logistics of collecting WB from a single donor are challenging but offer an alternative of reconstituting fresh blood components from different donors.[9] An international survey of cardiac programs performing congenital heart surgery in 2011 did not report any use of WB.[10]

Jobes and colleagues,[10] in 2015, described blood use in 4111 patients less than 2 years old who underwent elective cardiac surgery at the Children's Hospital of Philadelphia (CHOP) from 1995 to 2010, who standardly receive 2 units of fresh WB (collected <48 hours preoperatively) in the bypass prime and postoperatively in an institutional effort to reduce transfusions and donor exposure. Compared with published reports describing the use of blood components for comparable patient populations, children who received WB at CHOP had fewer donor exposures (median 2 donors, range 0–28) than patients who received standard blood components on the day of surgery and 1 day postoperatively.[10] The investigators hypothesize that fresh WB leads to a combination of increased function and number of platelets and increased coagulation factor levels, which contribute to improved hemostasis and less donor exposure. Although the investigators acknowledge an increasingly safe blood supply, they conclude that side effects, including transfusion-transmitted infection, which could result in lifelong sequelae, as well as parental concern are valid reasons to continue their practice of obtaining fresh WB.[10]

There is no consensus on the use of WB in pediatric cardiac surgery patients because the studies summarized earlier have conflicting conclusions, and differing blood product use, with some clinicians using WB for both CPB and postoperative transfusions and some for CPB only. Evidence suggests that pediatric patients who receive WB transfusions have decreased blood donor exposures. However, any further benefits of WB use in pediatric cardiac surgery are less clear and procurement of fresh WB continues to remain logistically challenging.

Use in Children Undergoing Craniofacial Surgery

In 2017, Thottathil and colleagues[5] retrospectively evaluated the use of WB (transfused within 3 days of collection) in the setting of pediatric complex cranial vault reconstruction surgery after the practice at CHOP changed from using reconstituted WB (RBCs and FFP) to the use of WB in 2013, in part because of its use in cardiovascular surgery at the same institution.[10] In a comparison of 59 children less than 4 years old who received reconstituted WB with 52 children who received WB, there was no difference in coagulation test abnormalities or thrombocytopenia postoperatively, although there was less donor exposure in the WB cohort (median 1 donor) versus the reconstituted WB cohort (median 2 donors) ($P = .02$). The investigators conclude that use of fresh WB is advantageous compared with component therapy because RBCs, clotting factors, and platelets are all delivered with only 1 donor exposure, although they caution that more study is needed.[5] Use of WB in this surgical setting needs further prospective study regarding the clinical benefits of its use compared with standard blood component therapy, which is more widely available.

Use in Pediatric Patients with Trauma

In 2018, Leeper and colleagues[3] prospectively compared 18 traumatically injured children more than 3 years of age weighing greater than 15 kg who received low-titer O WB (LTOWB) used within 14 days of collection with a historical cohort of 50 traumatically injured children who received standard blood products at 1 institution. The median time from emergency department admission to the start of LTOWB transfusion was 15 minutes (interquartile range [IQR], 14–77 minutes) versus 303 minutes (IQR, 129–741 minutes) for administration of at least 1 unit of RBCs, plasma, and platelets in the historical cohort ($P<.001$). There was no difference in laboratory markers of hemolysis, creatinine levels, or serum potassium levels between type O and non-type O patients, or in the LTOWB cohort compared with historical controls ($P>.38$). The investigators concluded that giving LTOWB to traumatically injured children was safe, although no clinical outcomes were compared, and that more research in larger cohorts of children is needed.[3]

In 2019, Leeper and colleagues[4] retrospectively compared 8 children 2 years of age and older who weighed at least 10 kg with severe trauma and resultant hemorrhagic shock who received LTOWB with 14 children who received conventional blood component therapy including conventional platelets at a single academic pediatric institution. The investigators noted no differences in posttransfusion platelet values and function via thromboelastography measurement of the maximum amplitude between the groups. Hospital mortality, intensive care unit (ICU) LOS, hospital LOS, and days on the ventilator were not significantly different between the groups (all P values >.20), although this small study was not powered to assess any difference in outcomes. Clearly, further prospective research is needed to assess the safety and efficacy of WB use in pediatric patients with trauma.

PATHOGEN-REDUCED BLOOD PRODUCTS

Pathogen reduction, or pathogen inactivation, are methods designed to treat blood components after collection such that broad categories of pathogens, including viruses, bacteria, and parasites, are neutralized by targeting their cell membranes, RNA, or DNA.[11] Some of the technologies for pathogen reduction also inactivate white blood cells, thus providing protection against transfusion-associated graft-versus-host disease, such as irradiation.[11]

Solvent/Detergent-Treated Plasma

Solvent/detergent-treated plasma (SDP) is a pooled product collected from more than 1000 donors who are screened for nonenveloped viruses, and extensively filtered to remove cells, cell fragments, and aggregates such that intracellular pathogens are effectively removed. The product is then treated with tri-N-butyl-phosphate for further pathogen and white blood cell inactivation. Subsequently, the product undergoes another round of sterile filtration such that bacteria and parasites are removed.[11] SDP has been licensed for use in Europe since the early 1990s and in the United States since 2013.[12,13] The package insert of Octoplas specifically states that it was evaluated in a prospective, open-label, single-arm, postmarketing study involving 50 pediatric patients (0–16 years old) and no hyperfibrinolytic or treatment-related thromboembolic events were noted,[14] and many European countries (Norway, Ireland, and Finland) use this product exclusively.[12]

In 2017, Camazine and colleagues[15] prospectively compared 357 children who received standard plasma (FFP or frozen plasma 24 [FP24]) with 62 who received SDP in 101 pediatric ICUs across 21 countries (**Table 2**). Patients were assigned based on the plasma transfusion practices of their local pediatric ICUs. There were no differences between the groups in patient age, gender, or illness severity, including pretransfusion International Normalized Ratio (INR) or reason for admission, although there was a significant difference for indication for plasma transfusion. Almost 36% of patients in the standard plasma arm were transfused without bleeding or a procedure, whereas almost 44% of patients in the SDP arm were transfused for minor bleeding ($P<.001$). There was no difference in posttransfusion INR reduction between the groups ($P = .8$). There was an independent reduction in mortality in the SDP group (14.5%) compared with the standard plasma group (29.1%) ($P = .02$) that persisted, although marginally ($P = .05$), when controlling for severity of illness, need for continuous renal replacement therapy, indication, and volume per kilogram of plasma product transfused. The investigators concluded that SDP use may be associated with improved survival but that more prospective, randomized clinical trials are needed to assess the safety and efficacy of SDP in critically ill children.[15]

INTERCEPT Platelets

An alternative strategy for pathogen reduction is through photochemical activation. The INTERCEPT blood system (Cerus Corporation, Concord, CA) uses amotosalen, a psoralen compound that binds to any available nucleic acids, inactivating both DNA and RNA viruses.[16] The blood product is then exposed to ultraviolet A light (wavelength 320–300 nm), which crosslinks amotosalen to the nucleic acid bases, therefore preventing replication and further pathogen reproduction. After the INTERCEPT treatment, an adsorption step removes the excess psoralen compound, leaving a very small quantity in the blood product.[16] The INTERCEPT system has been licensed in Europe since 2002, in the United States since 2014, and is the only photochemical activation platform approved by the Food and Drug Administration (FDA) as

Table 2
Studies of pathogen-reduced blood products in pediatrics

Reference	Patient Population Studied (n)	Blood Products Compared	Primary Outcome	Secondary Outcomes	Strengths	Caveats
Camazine et al,[15] 2017	Pediatric ICU patients who received plasma products (n = 419)	FFP/FP24 (n = 357) vs SDP (n = 62)	No difference in posttransfusion INR (P = .8)	Improvement in ICU mortality in SDP group (14%) compared with FFP/FP24 (29%) (P = .02)	Prospective, observational study	Assigned to receive each product based on local practice
Knutson et al,[19] 2015	Adults and pediatric patients in Europe. Pediatric patients <18 y old (n = 242 children; n = 46 neonates)	Platelets treated with INTERCEPT treatment compared with historical data on standard platelets	No severe adverse events with INTERCEPT platelets	Similar transfusion reaction rates to historical data with standard platelets and to adults. No adverse events, including skin rash, in neonates receiving concurrent phototherapy (n = 11)	—	Retrospective cohort study
Schulz et al,[20] 2019	Children aged 0–18 y who required platelet transfusion (n = 240 patients, n = 1932 transfusions)	Standard platelet transfusions (n = 860) vs PR platelet transfusions (n = 1072)	In patients 1–18 y old, difference seen in additional units of platelets needed in the 48 h following initial transfusion for PR platelets 1.4 units (SD ± 2.2) vs conventional 0.9 units (SD ± 1.6) (P<.001)	No difference in transfusion reactions	—	Retrospective cohort study

(continued on next page)

Table 2
(continued)

Reference	Patient Population Studied (n)	Blood Products Compared	Primary Outcome	Secondary Outcomes	Strengths	Caveats
Trakhtman et al,[24] 2016	Children <18 y old with cancer who required platelet transfusions (n = 137)	Mirasol-treated PR platelets (n = 51) compared with conventional platelets (n = 86)	No difference in the number of bleeding events, severity, and sites of bleeding between the 2 groups (P>.05 for all)	No difference in the rate of transfusion reactions in both groups. At 1–4 h posttransfusion, PR platelets had an increased CCI of 15.25 (SD ± 5.97) compared with standard platelets CCI 25.67 (SD ± 6.55) (P<.001), and 18–24 h post transfusion showed PR-platelet CCI 9.41 (SD ± 6.42) compared with standard platelets CCI 12.47 (SD ± 6.25) (P = .008)	—	Retrospective cohort study

| Jimenez-Marco et al,[25] 2019 | Children <15 y of age (n = 379), neonates in that cohort were separately evaluated (n = 132) | Neonates receiving Mirasol PR platelets (n = 132) compared with historical group who received conventional platelets (n = 99) | Patients who received PR platelets required mean 3.6 transfusions (SD ± 1.3) compared with conventional group required 1.8 transfusions (SD ± 0.8) (P = .031) | No increase in allergic transfusion reactions and no severe transfusion reactions | — | Single-center cohort study, used historical controls |

Abbreviations: CCI, corrected count index; FP24, frozen plasma 24; INR, International Normalized Ratio; PR, pathogen reduced.

of 2020.[12,17] There is an ongoing postmarketing surveillance study (the phase IV INTERCEPT Platelets Entering Routine use [PIPER] study) to evaluate the safety of transfusion of PR platelets in hematology/oncology patients, including pediatric patients.[18]

In 2015, Knutson and colleagues[19] prospectively reviewed 19,175 transfusions with INTERCEPT platelets in 4067 patients in Europe via an open-label, observational hemovigilance program at 21 centers in 11 European countries. Of these, 242 patients were less than 18 years of age, and 46 were neonates. No pediatric patients developed a severe adverse event related to the INTERCEPT platelets for at least 7 days posttransfusion, and they had a similar acute transfusion reaction rate (3.7%) to adults ($P = .179$).[19] No adverse events were reported in neonatal patients less than 28 days old (n = 46).[19] The investigators conclude that INTERCEPT platelets are well tolerated in patients, although the number of children in this study was small.

Schulz and colleagues[20] in 2019 performed a retrospective, single-center review of platelet usage in pediatric patients aged 0 to 18 years as part of a quality assurance program whereby 72 neonatal ICU (NICU) patients, 45 infants aged 0 to 12 months not admitted to the NICU, and 131 children aged 1 to 18 years received 1932 platelet transfusions of conventional platelets, PR platelets, or both as their institution transitioned from mainly conventional to mainly PR platelets. As a surrogate marker of efficacy in hemostasis, there were similar amounts of packed RBCs (pRBCs) transfused to patients over all age groups for clinically significant bleeding during the 48 hours after transfusion of both conventional and PR platelets. In patients 1 to 18 years old, there was a difference in additional platelet transfusions needed in the 48 hours following initial transfusion, with a mean of 1.4 subsequent platelet transfusions (standard deviation [SD] ± 2.2) for PR platelets versus mean of 0.9 transfusions (SD ± 1.6) for conventional platelets ($P<.001$).[20] A total of 10 allergic or febrile nonhemolytic transfusion reactions were reported, 6 out of 860 transfusions of conventional platelets (0.7%), and 4 out of 1072 transfusions of PR platelets (0.4%). Eleven neonates who received concurrent phototherapy and PR platelets were evaluated for skin rashes by an attending neonatologist because of the concern that the wavelengths from the phototherapy could interact with the psoralen product to cause a reaction, and none had a new rash. This finding is expected given that the optimal wavelength used in phototherapy to target neonatal unconjugated bilirubin is 460 to 490 nm, which is considerably more than the range of 300 to 320 nm used for the INTERCEPT system. The investigators concluded that their study supports the safety of PR platelet use in children.[20,21]

The Pathogen Inactivated Platelets use in Pediatric Patients: The International Experience (PIPPP) study is in progress to further study PR platelet use, safety, and efficacy in children in the United States and Europe given the small numbers of patients reported in all of the studies discussed earlier.[12]

Mirasol Platelets

Like other PR systems described earlier, the Mirasol system (Terumo BCT, Lakewood, CO) uses a photosensitizer compound (riboflavin) that is activated with ultraviolet B light. This compound then produces oxygen radicals, which irreversibly damages pathogens.[11] This technology has been licensed in Europe since 2007.[22] The FDA is awaiting results of a prospective, randomized controlled, noninferiority study to evaluate their clinical effectiveness in thrombocytopenic patients (including children) before licensure.[23]

In 2016, Trakhtman and colleagues[24] retrospectively compared 51 children with cancer who were randomly assigned to receive Mirasol PR platelets with 86 children who received conventional platelets. For the primary end point of proportion of patients with bleeding, there was no difference between the cohorts (28 patients had bleeding in the Mirasol group, and 40 patients had bleeding in the conventional group; $P = .29$). However, corrected count increments (CCIs), a secondary end point, differed between the 2 groups at 1 to 4 hours after transfusion, where patients who received PR platelets had a mean CCI of 15.25 (SD $\pm$ 5.97) and patients who received conventional platelets had a mean CCI of 25.67 (SD $\pm$ 6.55) ($P<.001$). At 18 to 24 hours after transfusion, patients receiving PR platelets had a mean CCI of 9.41 (SD $\pm$ 6.42), compared with a mean CCI of 12.47 (SD $\pm$ 6.25) in children who received conventional platelets ($P<.05$). All CCIs were greater than 7.5. The rate of transfusion-related adverse events was similar in both groups (8.3% in the Mirasol group vs 9.8% in the conventional group; $P = .73$). The investigators concluded that Mirasol PR platelets were efficacious for prophylactic use in pediatric oncology patients with thrombocytopenia.[24]

In 2019, Jimenez-Marco and colleagues[25] reported their experience transfusing Mirasol PR platelets in 379 children less than 15 years old after their center adopted universal use in 2013. Five children had transfusion reactions (1.32%), similar to the reaction rate in adults. In addition, they compared 132 neonates who received Mirasol PR platelets with a historical control group of 99 neonates who received conventional platelets. Neonates receiving the PR platelets required a mean of 3.6 platelet transfusions (SD $\pm$ 1.3), whereas neonates receiving conventional platelets required 1.8 transfusions (SD $\pm$ 0.3) ($P = .031$). The investigators concluded that PR platelets are safe for children; however, long-term and prospective studies are needed to further evaluate the safety and efficacy of PR platelets in children.[25]

FIBRINOGEN CONCENTRATE

Fibrinogen concentrate (FC) is produced from pooled plasma using the Cohn/Oncley cryoprecipitation procedure.[26] It then undergoes solvent/detergent exposure or pasteurization as a viral inactivation process for further reduction of pathogen transmission. Because of its production methods, it has a standardized fibrinogen concentration, which is advantageous compared with cryoprecipitate or FFP. The FDA approved the first FC product (RiaSTAP, CSL Behring, King of Prussia, PA) in the United States in 2009, and the second (Fibryna, Octapharma, Hoboken, NJ) in 2017.[27,28] Various forms of fibrinogen concentrations have been licensed for use in Brazil and Europe since the 1960s.[27] Pediatric studies of FC are summarized in **Table 3**.

Use in Children Undergoing Cardiac Surgery

In 2014, Galas and colleagues[29] performed a randomized prospective pilot study comparing 30 children less than 7 years old undergoing cardiac surgery with CPB with hypofibrinogenemia who received FC with 33 children who received cryoprecipitate. There was no difference in the primary outcome of the study, 48-hour postoperative blood loss with a median blood loss of 320 mL (IQR, 157–750 mL) in the FC cohort and 410 mL (IQR, 215–510 mL) in the cryoprecipitate cohort ($P = .672$).[29] There were no differences in secondary outcomes, including percentage of children exposed to allogeneic blood products perioperatively, duration of mechanical ventilation, vasopressor requirement, serious adverse event, ICU LOS stay, or death. The investigators concluded that FC is as effective and safe as cryoprecipitate in this patient population.[29]

Table 3
Studies of fibrinogen concentrate in pediatrics

Reference	Patient Population Studied (n)	Blood Products Compared	Primary Outcome	Secondary Outcomes	Strengths	Caveats
Galas et al,[29] 2014	Children <7 y of age undergoing cardiac surgery with CPB (n = 63)	60 mg/kg FC (n = 30) compared with 10 mL/kg cryoprecipitate (n = 33)	48-h postoperative blood loss in FC group 320 mL (IQR 157–750 mL) compared with cryoprecipitate 410 mL (IQR 215–510 mL) (P = .672)	No differences in percentage of children exposed to allogeneic blood products perioperatively, duration of mechanical ventilation, vasopressor requirement, serious adverse event, ICU LOS stay, or death	Prospective, randomized, blinded study	Single-center study
Massoumi et al,[30] 2018	Children <2 y of age who required nonemergent cardiac surgery with CPB (n = 90)	70 mg/kg of FC (n = 45) compared with 10 mL/kg of FFP (n = 45) post-CPB	Postoperative chest tube drainage more than first 24 h: 1.93 mL/kg/h (SD ± 6.63) vs 2.64 mL/kg/h (SD ± 2.18) (P = .04)	No difference in transfusion needs, postoperative complications, time of mechanical ventilation, ICU LOS, and inotrope support	Prospective, randomized study	Single-center study
Downey et al,[35] 2020	Children <12 mo of age who required nonemergent cardiac surgery with CPB (n = 60)	FC (n = 25) vs cryoprecipitate (n = 29) post-CPB	FC group required a median of 4 units of blood component (IQR 3–5) perioperatively vs cryoprecipitate group (5.5 units, IQR 4–7) (P = .01)	No differences in 24-h chest tube output, mechanical ventilation time, ICU LOS, and death	Prospective, randomized, 2 site study	—

| Giordano et al,[36] 2019 | Pediatric patients with ALL with hypofibrinogenemia (n = 101) | FC (n = 50) vs FFP (n = 51) | Mean time to normalization of fibrinogen levels: FC 1.6 d (±1 d) vs FFP 2 d (±1 d) (P = .04) | Proportion of patients with normalized fibrinogen levels: FC 94.4% vs FFP 67.1% (P = .04); no bleeding or thrombotic events reported | — | Retrospective cohort study |

Abbreviations: ALL, acute lymphoblastic leukemia; FC, fibrinogen concentrate.

In 2018, Massoumi and colleagues[30] performed a prospective, randomized, single-center study comparing 45 children less than 2 years old requiring nonemergent cardiac surgery requiring CPB who received FC with 45 children who received FFP for treatment of hypofibrinogenemic bleeding after bypass. Postoperative 24-hour chest tube drainage was less in the patients who received FC at 1.93 mL/kg/h (SD ± 6.63) compared with those who received FFP at 2.64 mL/kg/h (SD ± 2.18) (P = .04). There were no differences in postoperative transfusion needs, postoperative complications including need for return to surgery, ICU LOS, or inotrope support between the 2 groups. The investigators concluded that children in the FC arm received less pRBC support postoperatively (although not statistically less than children who received FFP) as a result of less bleeding, which they argue is clinically valuable given the independent association between pRBC transfusion and mortality and other poor outcomes.[30–34]

Downey and colleagues,[35] in 2020, performed a prospective, randomized controlled trial in the United States and compared 29 infants less than 12 months of age who underwent nonemergent cardiac surgery requiring CPB who received FC with 25 infants who received cryoprecipitate for hypofibrinogenemia after bypass. There was a significant difference between cohorts in the primary outcome of the study, which was exposure to allogeneic transfusion perioperatively. In the intention-to-treat analysis, infants treated with FC received a median of 4 intraoperative allogeneic units of blood components (IQR, 3–5 units) versus a median of 5.5 units (IQR, 4–7 units) in the cohort treated with cryoprecipitate. The infants treated with FC had a mean of 1.79 (95% confidence interval, 0.64–2.93; P = .003) fewer allogeneic blood donor exposures than the infants in the cryoprecipitate group. There were no differences in secondary outcomes, including 24-hour chest tube output, mechanical ventilation time, ICU LOS, and death within 30 days of surgery. The investigators concluded that FC is an acceptable alternative to cryoprecipitate when treating hypofibrinogenemia in infants after CPB.[35]

Use in Children with Acute Lymphoblastic Leukemia

In 2019, Giordano and colleagues[36] retrospectively reviewed the use of FC versus FFP in children with acute lymphoblastic leukemia (ALL) aged 1 to 18 years with severe hypofibrinogenemia after asparaginase administration. Children were treated at 15 medical centers in Italy, and treatment with FC or FFP differed based on local practice such that 50 children were treated with FC and 51 were treated with FFP. Children who received FC had faster normalization of fibrinogen levels (>70 mg/dL) compared with those who received FFP, with a mean time to normalization of fibrinogen levels of 1.6 ± 1 days compared with 2 ± 1 days in the plasma group (P = .04). There was also a greater proportion of patients who subsequently achieved normal fibrinogen levels (>70 mg/dL) in the FC cohort compared with those who received FFP (94.4% vs 67.1%; P = .04), although fibrinogen level before treatment was also independently associated with normalization in multivariate analysis. There were no severe reactions, significant bleeding, or thrombotic complications in either group. The investigators concluded that FC was safe and effective for treatment of hypofibrinogenemia in children with ALL, although prospective studies including its cost-effectiveness compared with plasma are needed.[36]

SUMMARY

This article describes the most current and relevant studies of novel blood component therapy use in children, including WB, SDP, PR platelets, and FC. Although limited data are available on the safety and efficacy of these novel blood components in pediatric patients, wider use is expected in this vulnerable population, especially because all these therapies are licensed for use in children in Europe, the United States, and other countries. In addition, there are some novel blood components that have not been studied for use at all in children, including PR WB and RBCs, cold stored platelets, freeze-dried plasma, and hemoglobin-based oxygen carriers. Given the continued paucity of prospective, rigorous studies designed specifically to study the use of new products in children, it is critical that treating physicians and the pediatric transfusion medicine community continue to appraise best evidence for their use and advocate pediatric patient inclusion in random clinical trials and prospective observational trials.

DISCLOSURE

The authors have nothing to disclose.

REFERENCES

1. Spinella PC, Cap AP. Whole blood: back to the future. Curr Opin Hematol 2016; 23(6):536–42.
2. Manno CS, Hedberg KW, Kim HC, et al. Comparison of the hemostatic effects of fresh whole blood, stored whole blood, and components after open heart surgery in children. Blood 1991;77(5):930–6.
3. Leeper CM, Yazer MH, Cladis FP, et al. Use of uncrossmatched cold-stored whole blood in injured children with hemorrhagic shock. JAMA Pediatr 2018;172(5): 491–2.
4. Leeper CM, Yazer MH, Cladis FP, et al. Cold-stored whole blood platelet function is preserved in injured children with hemorrhagic shock. J Trauma Acute Care Surg 2019;87(1):49–53.
5. Thottathil P, Sesok-Pizzini D, Taylor JA, et al. Whole blood in pediatric craniofacial reconstruction surgery. J Craniofac Surg 2017;28(5):1175–8.
6. Groom RC, Froebe S, Martin J, et al. Update on pediatric perfusion practice in North America: 2005 survey. J Extra Corpor Technol 2005;37(4):343–50.
7. Mou SS, Giroir BP, Molitor-Kirsch EA, et al. Fresh whole blood versus reconstituted blood for pump priming in heart surgery in infants. N Engl J Med 2004; 351(16):1635–44.
8. Valleley MS, Buckley KW, Hayes KM, et al. Are there benefits to a fresh whole blood vs. packed red blood cell cardiopulmonary bypass prime on outcomes in neonatal and pediatric cardiac surgery? J Extra Corpor Technol 2007;39(3): 168–76.
9. Gruenwald CE, McCrindle BW, Crawford-Lean L, et al. Reconstituted fresh whole blood improves clinical outcomes compared with stored component blood therapy for neonates undergoing cardiopulmonary bypass for cardiac surgery: a randomized controlled trial. J Thorac Cardiovasc Surg 2008;136(6):1442–9.
10. Jobes DR, Sesok-Pizzini D, Friedman D. Reduced transfusion requirement with use of fresh whole blood in pediatric cardiac surgical procedures. Ann Thorac Surg 2015;99(5):1706–11.
11. Stramer SL, Galel SA. Infectious disease screening. In: Fung MK, Eder AF, Spitaknik SL, et al, editors. Technical Manual. 19th ed. Bethesda, MD: American Association of Blood Banks; 2017. p. 161–205.
12. Jacquot C, Delaney M. Pathogen-inactivated blood products for pediatric patients: blood safety, patient safety, or both? Transfusion 2018;58(9):2095–101.

13. "Octaplas pediatric approval". US Food and Drug administration. 2019. Available at: https://www.fda.gov/media/123133/download. Accessed August 27, 2020.

14. Octaplas [package insert]. Hoboken (NJ): Octapharma; 2019.

15. Camazine MN, Karam O, Colvin R, et al. Outcomes related to the use of frozen plasma or pooled solvent/detergent-treated plasma in critically ill children. Pediatr Crit Care Med 2017;18(5):e215–23.

16. Intercept blood system platelet [package insert]. Concord (CA): Cerus Corporation; 2019.

17. Lu W, Fung M. Platelets treated with pathogen reduction technology: current status and future direction. F1000Res 2020;9:F1000.

18. Cerus Corporation. An open label, post-marketing surveillance study following transfusion of INTERCEPT platelet components (PIPER). (Identifier NCT02549222). 2015. Available at: https://clinicaltrials.gov/ct2/show/NCT02549222. Accessed August 27, 2020.

19. Knutson F, Osselaer J, Pierelli L, et al. A prospective, active haemovigilance study with combined cohort analysis of 19,175 transfusions of platelet components prepared with amotosalen-UVA photochemical treatment. Vox Sang 2015;109(4):343–52.

20. Schulz WL, McPadden J, Gehrie EA, et al. Blood utilization and transfusion reactions in pediatric patients transfused with conventional or pathogen reduced platelets. J Pediatr 2019;209:220–5.

21. Bhutani VK, Committee on Fetus and Newborn, American Academy of Pediatrics. Phototherapy to prevent severe neonatal hyperbilirubinemia in the newborn infant 35 or more weeks of gestation. Pediatrics 2011;128(4):e1046–52.

22. "The right path to advancing blood safety: safe, simple, effective." Mirasol® pathogen reduction technology. Available at: www.terumobct.com/mirasol. Accessed August 31, 2020.

23. Terumo BCTbio. Efficacy of mirasol-treated apheresis platelets in patients with hypoproliferative thrombocytopenia (MIPLATE). (Identifier: NCT02964325). 2016. Available at: https://clinicaltrials.gov/ct2/show/NCT02964325. Accessed August 27, 2020.

24. Trakhtman P, Karpova O, Balashov D, et al. Efficacy and safety of pathogen-reduced platelet concentrates in children with cancer: a retrospective cohort study. Transfusion 2016;56(Suppl 1):S24–8.

25. Jimenez-Marco T, Garcia-Recio M, Girona-Llobera E. Use and safety of riboflavin and UV light-treated platelet transfusions in children over a five-year period: focusing on neonates. Transfusion 2019;59(12):3580–8.

26. Franchini M, Lippi G. Fibrinogen replacement therapy: a critical review of the literature. Blood Transfus 2012;10(1):23–7.

27. Costa-Filho R, Hochleitner G, Wendt M, et al. Over 50 Years of fibrinogen concentrate. Clin Appl Thromb Hemost 2016;22(2):109–14.

28. "FDA approves Fibryna". US Food and Drug administration. 2017. Available at: https://www.fda.gov/media/105873/download. Accessed August 27, 2020.

29. Galas FR, de Almeida JP, Fukushima JT, et al. Hemostatic effects of fibrinogen concentrate compared with cryoprecipitate in children after cardiac surgery: a randomized pilot trial. J Thorac Cardiovasc Surg 2014;148(4):1647–55.

30. Massoumi G, Mardani D, Mousavian SM, et al. Comparison of the effect of fibrinogen concentrate with fresh frozen plasma (FFP) in management of hypofibrinogenemic bleeding after congenital cardiac surgeries: a clinical trial study. ARYA Atheroscler 2018;14(6):248–53.

31. Salvin JW, Scheurer MA, Laussen PC, et al. Blood transfusion after pediatric cardiac surgery is associated with prolonged hospital stay. Ann Thorac Surg 2011; 91(1):204–10.
32. Kipps AK, Wypij D, Thiagarajan RR, et al. Blood transfusion is associated with prolonged duration of mechanical ventilation in infants undergoing reparative cardiac surgery. Pediatr Crit Care Med 2011;12(1):52–6.
33. Iyengar A, Scipione CN, Sheth P, et al. Association of complications with blood transfusions in pediatric cardiac surgery patients. Ann Thorac Surg 2013;96(3): 910–6.
34. Wolf MJ, Maher KO, Kanter KR, et al. Early postoperative bleeding is independently associated with increased surgical mortality in infants after cardiopulmonary bypass. J Thorac Cardiovasc Surg 2014;148(2):631–6.e1.
35. Downey LA, Andrews J, Hedlin H, et al. Fibrinogen concentrate as an alternative to cryoprecipitate in a postcardiopulmonary transfusion algorithm in infants undergoing cardiac surgery: a prospective randomized controlled trial. Anesth Analg 2020;130(3):740–51.
36. Giordano P, Grassi M, Saracco P, et al. Human fibrinogen concentrate and fresh frozen plasma in the management of severe acquired hypofibrinogenemia in children with acute lymphoblastic leukemia: results of a retrospective survey. J Pediatr Hematol Oncol 2019;41(4):275–9.

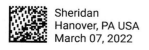